D0742028

Preventing Preterm Birth: A Parent's Guide

Michael Katz, Pamela Gill, Judith Turiel
Editors

Health Publishing Company
A division of Northern California Medical Services, Inc.
(In affiliation with Children's Hospital of San Francisco)
3700 California Street
San Francisco, California 94118

© 1988 Michael Katz, M.D., Pamela Gill, R.N., Judith Turiel, Ed.D.
All rights reserved

8 7 6 5 4 3 2 1

Editing and Production Coordination: Nancy Adess Editing
Cover and book design: Kristin Prentice, Sphinx Graphics
Illustrations: Felicia Noëlle Trujillo
Typesetting: Judy Lambert

Printed in the United States of America

Library of Congress Catalog Card No. 87-83554

ISBN 0-931421-11-X

Preventing

Preterm

Birth:

A

Parent's

Guide

EDITORS:
Michael Katz, M.D.
Pamela Gill, R.N., M.S.N.
Judith Turiel, Ed.D.

This book was a cooperative effort of the following people:
Nancy Adler, Ph.D.
Gloria Levine Bryant, M.A.
Kendal Bryant, Ph.D.
Pamela Gill, R.N., M.S.N.
Michael Katz, M.D.
Gail Nethercutt, Ph.D.
Sally Sehring, M.D.
Shari Ser, R.P.T.
Meg Stern
Judith Turiel, Ed.D.

Health Publishing Company
A division of Northern California Medical Services, Inc.
In affiliation with Children's Hospital of San Francisco

To all the
would-be premature babies
and all the mothers and fathers
who experienced preterm labor.
One of the greatest gifts
in a child's life
is a healthy
start.

Table
of
Contents

33

Self-Monitoring for Preterm Labor

What Are the Signs and Symptoms of Preterm Labor?
How to Monitor
When to Monitor
What to Do if You Detect Frequent or Regular
Uterine Tightening

CHAPTER

The Diagnosis of Preterm Labor

CHAPTER

Bedrest at Home

Medical Home Visits
Feelings: Some Good, Some Bad
Getting Organized at Home
How to Eat Well When You Must Rest in Bed

CHAPTER

Cerclage

CHAPTER

7

Tocolytic Medications

Beta-Adrenergic Medications
Magnesium Sulfate
Other Substances
When Tocolytic Medications Should *Not* Be Used

List of Illustrations

INTRODUCTION

As you pick up this book, you may be pregnant, the partner of a pregnant woman, or thinking about a future pregnancy. You may know that you face an "increased risk" of delivering your baby before the full nine months, or you may just be wondering whether you will have any problems. Every pregnant woman hopes for a normal, easy pregnancy and a healthy baby. At the same time, most women have some concerns about problems that can arise.

This book provides current information about the problem of preterm labor and delivery, and about ways to minimize the most serious consequences of this problem. Fortunately, there are steps that you and your doctor can take to increase the likelihood that you will have a healthy baby. This book explains these steps. It is a guide to help you through your months of pregnancy if you have a higher-than-average risk for a premature delivery. It should be used in conjunction with experienced obstetric care.

At present, medical science can predict about one-half of all premature deliveries by looking for certain signs or by considering a woman's medical history. But 50 percent of prematurely born infants are born to mothers who do not have any of the risk factors known to be associated with preterm birth (*described in Chapter One*). Unfortunately, we are not able to alert these women ahead of time about taking some extra precautions.

We think *any* pregnant woman can benefit from the information provided in this book. However, it is designed especially for those of you whose past and/or present situation suggests an increased chance of preterm labor—you are among the 50 percent we *can* help. By knowing that your pregnancy is considered "high risk," you and your medical care providers can increase awareness, precaution, and careful observation during your pregnancy. If preterm labor does develop, it can be diagnosed early, in time for proper treatment to give you the best chances of carrying your baby to term.

Why Is Preterm Labor a Serious Concern?

In spite of major improvements in medical care for pregnant women and their newborn babies, prematurity remains the number one problem in today's obstetric care. Prematurity is responsible for more than 85 percent of the deaths among newborn infants in the United States, and is a major cause of illness and developmental problems among newborns who survive the first month after birth. Simply put, preterm labor is a serious concern because it can have so great an impact on the life and well-being of babies and their families.

Traditionally, medical care has placed very little emphasis on *prevention* of preterm births. The focus has been mainly on treating premature infants *after* they are born. Sophisticated, highly technological intensive-care nurseries have been built, and have helped many sick babies. As a result, many very premature babies now survive who would have died without such care.

However, many of these "survivors" face serious medical complications that can last for months, years, or throughout life. Even the newest intensive care nurseries cannot solve the complex problems associated with very premature births—problems involving the health of the premature infant and the emotional and physical burden on parents, as well as the expense placed on families and on society as a whole. In addition, this treatment raises serious ethical dilemmas for individual families and society, since success in ensuring the survival of infants born more and more prematurely results in more and more infants who are severely damaged, perhaps for life.

A New Approach

In recent years, medical care has increasingly emphasized *preventing* premature births. The goal is to help a pregnancy last longer, and get closer to full term, in order to improve chances for a healthy, normal baby. The underlying view is simple: The best place for most developing preterm babies is inside the mother's womb.

Although medications that can stop the contractions of preterm labor have been available for many years, these medications are successful only if started *early* in a woman's preterm labor. Unfortunately, however, most women who experience preterm labor arrive at the hospital or doctor's office too late for effective treatment to stop that labor. In other words, a *preventive* approach depends upon *early diagnosis and treatment* of preterm labor.

As a result, medical teams are developing a new kind of prenatal care for women who are "at risk" for preterm labor— the kind of care described in this book. Of course, the basics of good prenatal care are essential, including adequate nutrition, rest, avoidance of harmful substances, and regular visits to a health professional who can check the health of the fetus and mother-to-be. If your pregnancy is high risk, however, you also need information and training that will help you participate actively in managing your pregnancy. Your role in your own prenatal care can include *early discovery* of irregularities that may be preterm labor.

Given our present knowledge, there is no way to prevent preterm labor. Early discovery of preterm *labor*, however, may stop it from progressing to preterm *delivery*. This book helps you learn to detect early signs of preterm labor. It teaches you how to monitor your own uterine activity throughout your pregnancy, and to recognize other subtle signs of preterm labor. In addition, it explains when you should alert your ob/gyn or other practitioner, who can then examine you to see whether preterm labor has indeed begun.

Our experience using this approach at one San Francisco hospital has been encouraging. Before setting up a program to train high-risk pregnant women (and partners) to monitor uterine activity, we could stop preterm labor in only about 25 percent of the women who had it. Among women who participated in the new educational program, more than 90 percent who experienced preterm labor were treated effectively to stop the labor. In the great majority of these women, the pregnancy then lasted close to nine months.

As you read this book, keep in mind that many precautions you can take during pregnancy involve your own monitoring for unusual signs, and perhaps some easing of daily activities. More aggressive medical treatments should be given only when they appear to be necessary *in your case*.

What this book includes:

- **Description of actions you can take to monitor your pregnancy and to lessen possible problems by discovering them early.**

- **Medical information about diagnosis and treatment of preterm labor, and about the premature infant.**

- **Discussion of the experience of preterm labor—in case you do face this condition—and of decisions that may arise during medical treatment.**

- **Suggestions of ways you might cope, physically and emotionally, with the sometimes difficult days at various stages of a "high-risk" pregnancy.**

What this book is not:

- **This book is not a basic guide to pregnancy—for example, nutritional needs and other aspects of basic prenatal care. Many books and pamphlets are available in bookstores and libraries on this subject. Ask your doctor, nurse, or librarian.**

- **This book is not a "prescription" for your care or treatment. Every woman's pregnancy is different and should be treated according to her specific needs.**

- **And finally, this book is not a guarantee that you can avoid a preterm delivery. Sometimes preterm labor may occur despite efforts of you and your provider. If you do have a preterm delivery, appropriate, immediate care in a neonatal intensive-care nursery brings good chances for a happy outcome.**

About the Authors

This book is written by a medical and consumer team working with Children's Hospital of San Francisco. The team includes: a doctor and a nurse who specialize in high-risk obstetric care; a neonatologist experienced in caring for premature infants; psychologists working on health issues; a physical therapist; a woman who develops special exercise programs; a consumer-health educator who twice experienced preterm labor—delivering a healthy baby boy following the "preventive" approach; and a new mother and father whose healthy baby girl was born after extended hospital treatment to stop preterm labor.

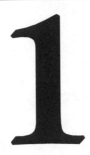

What Is
Preterm
Labor?

The length of pregnancy is figured by counting the weeks since the date of your last menstrual period (LMP). Although most people think of a full-term pregnancy simply as nine months long, the definition of "term" delivery is: *delivery after 37 weeks since your last menstrual period.* If delivery occurs between 20 and 36 weeks of pregnancy, it is called a *preterm delivery (see figure 1).* (For the many women who do not have regularly spaced periods, special calculations are made to determine the length of pregnancy.) As you will see, knowing the number of weeks of your pregnancy may be very important if signs of an early labor seem to occur.

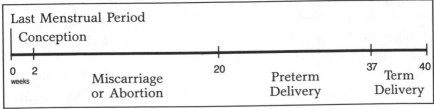

Figure 1 — Stages of pregnancy.

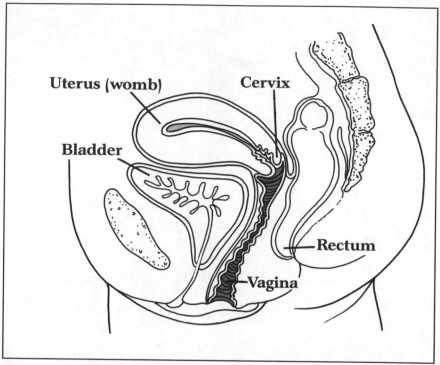

Figure 2 — Uterus and cervix during pregnancy.

The process that brings about delivery of the baby is called *labor.* "Going into labor" is characterized by: 1) *uterine activity* (most commonly known as uterine contractions, or contractions of the womb); and 2) opening and shortening of the *cervix* (the bottom segment of the uterus, *see figure 2*). When this combination of events occurs before 37 weeks of pregnancy, it is considered *preterm labor.* If not stopped, preterm labor will ultimately result in a *preterm delivery.*

Most women have some uterine contractions before the 37th week of pregnancy. Such contractions are normal. This book is most concerned about *excessive* uterine activity *that is combined with changes in the cervix.* The following chapters will teach you how to distinguish between normal and excessive uterine activity; however, only your health care provider can check for cervical changes.

You are the person closest to your uterus at all times and, with training, you can help detect preterm labor in its early stages. With early detection of preterm labor, effective treatment is more likely. Effective treatment means prolonging the pregnancy through crucial weeks of a baby's growth before birth.

Who Is At Risk for Developing Preterm Labor? And What Does "At Risk" Mean?

Between six and 10 of every 100 pregnant women will have a premature baby. In a group of 100 pregnant women, however, some individuals have a greater chance than others of delivering early. We cannot predict with great accuracy which women will develop preterm labor and when this will happen, because the causes of labor—whether at term or early—remain unknown.

Nevertheless, experience has helped identify certain conditions that can lead to preterm labor and delivering a preterm baby. Women who have one or more of these conditions are often referred to as *high risk*. Keep in mind, however, that being "at risk" does *not* mean that you *will* experience preterm labor or delivery. It means that you and your health care provider should watch very carefully for early signs of preterm labor in case it does develop. In some cases, these conditions can be corrected. For example, an infection of the urinary tract and kidneys during pregnancy is thought to increase the risk of preterm labor and delivery significantly. If the infection is diagnosed and treated, however, the risk will be reduced.

What Are These "At Risk" Conditions?

A number of conditions, or *risk factors*, have been associated with an increased incidence of preterm labor and delivery (*see figure 3*).

So What Are My Odds?

About 10 to 15 of every 100 pregnant women have one or more of the risk factors listed in figure 3. Of these high-risk women, approximately 20 to 30 percent will actually develop preterm labor—that is, about three or four of our original 100 pregnant women (*see figure 4*). For most of these conditions, therefore, it is more likely that preterm labor will *not* develop than that it will. Nevertheless, it is wise to

Risk Factors Associated With Preterm Labor

Major Factors

1. Previous preterm labor or delivery
2. Misshapen uterus
3. DES daughter
4. Abdominal surgery and/or cerclage
5. More than two second-trimester abortions (spontaneous or therapeutic
6. Cone biopsy
7. Multiple pregnancy: twins, triplets, etc.
8. Cervical change and/or excessive uterine contractions at less than 33 weeks of pregnancy
9. Serious infection during this pregnancy
10. Excessive amount of amniotic fluid
11. Unexplained vaginal bleeding after 20 weeks of pregnancy

Minor Factors

1. More than two first-trimester abortions (spontaneous or therapeutic
2. Bleeding after the first 12 weeks of pregnancy
3. Urinary tract infection during this pregnancy
4. Smoking more than 10 cigarettes per day
5. Extreme mental or physical stress

Figure 3 — Risk factors associated with preterm labor.

be alert to possible problems, and by following some of the guidelines in this book, you can reduce the odds of preterm birth even more.

Preterm and Premature

Although some babies born one or two weeks before the 37-week "term" are healthy enough not to need special medical care, most preterm babies are also premature in their development. *Maturity* refers to the baby's ability to live outside the womb, while *term* refers to a certain length of time since your last menstrual period. Any baby who has not reached full

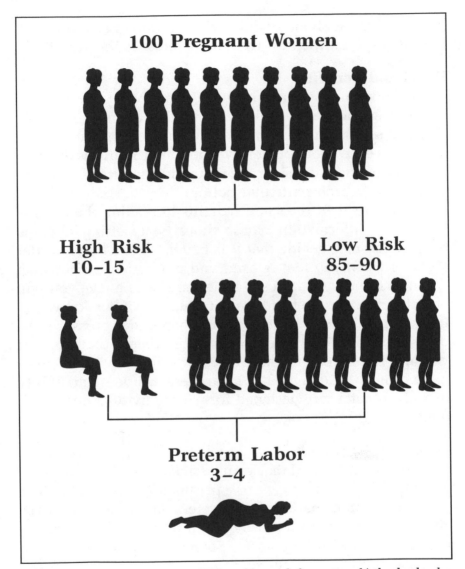

Figure 4 — Number of women at high and low risk for preterm birth who develop preterm labor.

maturity by the time of birth—whether born early or at term—needs to stay in the neonatal intensive-care nursery until she or he reaches functional maturity.

Chapter Nine describes in greater detail a baby's development at different stages of pregnancy. For now, keep in mind that every week gained during your pregnancy increases your baby's maturity. As you approach 37 weeks and beyond, you increase the likelihood of delivering a *mature* baby who will not need special medical treatments outside the womb.*

Risks and Benefits

An important step in making decisions about preterm labor is the weighing of risks and benefits. Throughout this book, you will see that any recommendation about medical treatment, and even about preventive measures, requires that you and your provider consider the risks and benefits for you and your baby of each particular action.

There are even risks and benefits to reading this book— some of the information may, at times, be upsetting for some people. You may decide that it is better to read these harder sections when you feel relaxed and unworried, rather than when you're nervous. Despite the risks, we believe you will be better prepared to handle most situations if you know and think about them *beforehand* rather than under pressure. We think the risk of increased concern or anxiety that some of you may feel in reading this book is worth the overall benefit to be gained through greater awareness, caution, and ability to seek prenatal care designed for your individual needs. We hope you agree!

A Developing Field

It is very important that your prenatal care provider is experienced in handling *high-risk* pregnancies, and is familiar with current information about preterm labor. If you find our suggestions differ from those of your provider, talk over the pros and cons with him or her. Sometimes, you may wish to get another opinion about recommended treatments—a desire your provider should support.

In using this book, keep in mind that management of high-risk pregnancies is a developing field. Sometimes, there is no

Spontaneous and Indicated Preterm Deliveries. In some pregnancies (less than 20 percent of all preterm births) babies must be delivered before 37 weeks because of disease in the mother or baby. For example, a pregnant woman may have dangerously high blood pressure or there may be signs of problems with the fetus that are better treated outside the womb. In such cases, preterm delivery occurs intentionally, either by inducing labor with drugs or by a cesarean section operation. This type of preterm delivery is called an *indicated preterm delivery*—that is, it is indicated by disease in the mother and/or baby. These deliveries, of course, cannot be prevented by the type of monitoring described in this book. In contrast, *spontaneous preterm deliveries* are those which result from preterm labor which progressed to a delivery. This type of delivery is the concern of this book.

single "right answer." Health care providers do disagree on certain aspects of diagnosis and treatment. Individual doctors may differ in their interpretation of information and their judgments about medical treatments. Also, knowledge and practice change over time.

Prevention of preterm birth requires attention and resources at many levels. With improved living conditions, education, and better nutrition, fewer women will be at risk for pregnancy problems and will need less medical intervention. At the same time, we can all contribute to making the medical approach safer and more effective when it is needed. Informed patients are important for reaching that goal.

Your Role in Reaching Decisions

Throughout this book, we try to provide basic information that can help you be actively involved in decisions about your pregnancy. We emphasize the need to consider risks and benefits—pros and cons—for any medical intervention, as well as for no or minimal treatment. Appropriate care requires educated judgments about the likely outcomes for mother and baby. There are no "cookbook" steps that can be followed in every case of high-risk pregnancy, because every woman and every pregnancy are different. As you learn about choices and considerations that relate to your circumstances, you may want to write down advantages, disadvantages, and questions you have about decisions in your own case—and talk these over with your health care providers.

For many decisions, your common sense and personal priorities are often needed to evaluate the pros and cons. At other times you may need to rely more on the knowledge and experience of your health care providers—a reminder of how important it is to choose carefully (*see Chapter Two*).

Remember also that in many situations, there is time— and it is certainly acceptable—to obtain a second opinion from another experienced practitioner about a recommended treatment.

There may be times when you just do not feel up to having a very active involvement in a complex medical decision. You may want to step back and let your health care provider make the judgment. Don't be surprised by this need—it is perfectly understandable and normal; you are the best judge of how much involvement you want and when you want it. Your role does not need to be an all-or-nothing proposition. Trust your instincts about what feels comfortable for you at different times. Talk openly with your practitioner, and let her or him know when you want more—or less—involvement.

Similar considerations hold true for the decision-making role of your partner, relatives, and friends. A supportive partner can be a great help in reaching decisions during pregnancy and the process of labor and delivery. Depending on individual circumstances, however, there may be times when involvement of others does not feel helpful. Again, there are no rules—each woman should decide when and to what extent she wants and needs the participation of her partner, family, or friends. If difficulties or tensions develop over involvement of a particular person, you may wish to talk with your doctor, nurse, or a social worker.

Living Your Life While Pregnant: Questions and Answers

Q: *I've just read this book's introductory section. I am now aware that I fit into one of the categories associated with increased incidence of preterm labor, but that this does not mean I will face this problem. Does my entire pregnancy have to be different because I am at higher risk for preterm labor, even if I have no signs of unusual contractions?*

A: You should live your life as normally as possible throughout your pregnancy, even though you are considered at risk for preterm labor. Before turning to special recommendations for your pregnancy, let's review common changes of pregnancy:

- **increased weight**

- **metabolic changes**

- **bodily changes as baby grows**

- **fatigue**

- **mood swings or "feeling emotional"**

Although some women seem to live and work as always, up to the day they deliver, most women do modify their activities in some way—take daily naps, reduce or stop work toward the end of pregnancy, change diet and drinking habits, cut down on physical activity. All women should receive regular prenatal care throughout pregnancy. They should be aware of the physical changes of their own body and, particularly, of the presence of excessive uterine contractions (*see Chapter Three*). A woman at risk for preterm labor should also do the following:

✔ **Check her uterus by feeling for contractions during daily activities, to detect irregularities and to learn what activities may need to be modified.**

✔ **Work a bit more closely with her prenatal health care providers, and be sure to keep them informed about how she is feeling.**

We discuss both of these activities more fully in later chapters.

Q: *Is there a way I can prevent preterm labor?*

A: Unfortunately, we cannot identify a treatment or give a recommendation that will prevent preterm labor. Therefore, we try to prevent preterm *births* by detecting labor in its early stages, and by learning what factors may be associated with the beginning of those first stages of preterm labor. If these factors in a woman's life can be modified during her pregnancy, her chances of experiencing preterm labor may be reduced. Among the general factors presently associated with the onset of preterm labor are:

- **stress**

- **fatigue**

- **long or exhausting travel**
- **poor nutrition**
- **unusual physical activity**

Since every woman is an individual, she needs to learn whether particular activities are associated with increased uterine contractions *in her case.*

Often, there is no identifiable reason for the start of preterm labor. Even with changes in lifestyle during pregnancy, there are times when preterm labor cannot be prevented. However, if preterm labor is identified early—with careful monitoring and awareness by you and your provider—preterm *delivery* can usually be prevented or delayed, giving your baby crucial extra time to grow.

Q: *Should I stay in bed during my pregnancy?*

A: There is presently no evidence that staying on bedrest during any particular weeks of pregnancy will prevent preterm labor or a preterm birth. Lying down for a while during the day, if this can be arranged, may help the problem of fatigue. For some women who do begin showing unusual uterine activity or changes in the cervix, bedrest may be recommended as a "first line of defense." Also, women who are diagnosed and treated for preterm labor will spend some time on bedrest. We discuss the special considerations for these women in Chapter Five.

Q: *I work outside the home and want to continue during my pregnancy. Also, I need the income. Will this be a problem?*

A: Women who are at high risk for preterm delivery do not usually need to stop working unless preterm labor is actually diagnosed. If your job is very strenuous—for example, involving much lifting or other physical activity—you should talk this over with your obstetrician. The following suggestions may make your job easier on your pregnancy, and perhaps allow you to stay at work longer.

- **Try to schedule rest times throughout the day and find a place to lie down** (perhaps you will need to bring a small cot).

- **Avoid a full bladder; make frequent trips to the rest room.**

- **Monitor for uterine contractions while at work to see whether certain aspects of your job cause increased uterine activity.** (You can monitor while sitting or standing.)

- **Try not to let things bother you or cause anxiety, even if they normally would; for those months, see if you can detach yourself from the usual stresses of your job.**

- **Find out about disability coverage from your company and/or state for the time when you do stop working.**

Q: *How much physical exercise should I do if I am* not *having excessive uterine activity or cervical changes?*

A: A general rule of thumb is to avoid *new* kinds of exercise during your pregnancy. That is, don't start playing tennis or taking aerobics classes if you were not already used to it. When you do exercise, monitor for uterine contractions during and after; if the exercise is causing problems, you may need to cut back or stop. Many providers think high-risk women should avoid running and activities such as weight-lifting, horseback riding, or other very strenuous or jarring exercise. Describe to your practitioner the kind and amount of exercise you normally do, and see whether she or he thinks changes are necessary.

Q: *I'm planning to take a prenatal childbirth class, such as Lamaze. Is there any reason I can't do this? How about general prenatal exercise classes?*

A: Each woman needs to decide how cautious she wants to be, and should also discuss exercise programs with her obstetrician. There is no reason you cannot join childbirth or other exercise classes, if your practitioner agrees it is safe. However, you should be very careful about monitoring for any activities that cause you to have contractions, and avoid those particular activities. In general, it is probably wise to sit out those exercises that put pressure on your abdomen or that have you bearing down or stretching the cervix. Also, you should *not* rub or stimulate your nipples before 36 weeks as this stimulation can lead to uterine contractions.

If you do develop excessive uterine contractions and/or cervical changes, you will need to limit your physical activity and change the type of exercise you are doing. And again, your individual exercise program and limits should be worked out with your practitioner.

Q: *Is it okay for me to have sexual intercourse during pregnancy?*

A: There is no definite answer to this question. In some women, intercourse appears to initiate preterm labor, while in others it does not. Orgasm in women does involve contractions of the uterus; however, in most women who are pregnant, these contractions do stop rather than develop into preterm labor. We suggest you discuss this question with your partner and practitioner, so that you can work out an answer that is appropriate and comfortable for your pregnancy. (Speaking of comfort and caution: As your pregnancy progresses, the safest position is probably woman-on-top.)

A related concern involves sexual desire or interest during pregnancy. In any pregnancy, the woman's interest varies; about the same proportion of women report increased interest, decreased interest, or no change. For women who are aware of their risk for preterm delivery, it is very common to shy away from sexual intercourse. Concern about the possibility of causing problems is enough to dampen sexual desires and activity. If you experience such a reaction, rest assured—it is completely normal! Again, it will probably help to talk with your partner about these concerns.

Q: *You say stress is associated with the onset of preterm labor—What do you mean by "stress?" Sometimes I just feel upset about the whole thing, other times I feel better.*

A: The definition of "stress" is very fuzzy. What is stressful for one person is not for another (*see figure 5*). What is stressful one day may not be stressful to the same person a day later. You are absolutely right that being at risk or experiencing preterm labor can be upsetting at times or cause stress. Many women feel better knowing they can lower the chance of serious problems by carefully monitoring their own pregnancy and working closely with their health care providers. Also,

---

Climbing stairs

Driving a car

Taking public transportation

Fatigue
At home
At work

Full bladder
(including at work)

Poor nutrition
(including alcohol, harmful substances)

Urinary/vaginal infection

Constipation

Sexual intercourse/orgasm

Breast stimulation

Travel

Prenatal exercise classes

Figure 5 — Activities and other factors associated with onset of preterm labor in some women. Think about ways to minimize those that seem to cause problems for you.

some women are able to identify and alter certain aspects of their lives—at home, at work, in dealing with people—that generally cause them to feel stress or anxiety. You may find it helpful to talk with other women who have been through a high-risk pregnancy, or with an experienced professional (such as a hospital social worker or an obstetric nurse).

Q: *Is there a time period when I need to be particularly cautious, or are all of the weeks pretty much the same?*

A: Although every week of pregnancy is important for your baby's development, there is a stretch of time, between 25 and 30 weeks' gestation, when you may want to be particularly cautious about possible preterm labor. A baby born during those weeks will spend much time in the intensive-care nursery, and is likely to experience serious problems relating to prematurity. The long-term outcome for such an infant is uncertain (*see Chapter Nine*). It is very important to try to get beyond these weeks, closer to a full-term pregnancy.

CHAPTER

2

Prenatal
Care:
Choosing an
Obstetrician
and a
Pediatrician

A preventive approach to
preterm birth is a team approach. You and your prenatal care
provider are the central team members. Your provider needs
to be trained and experienced in handling high-risk pregnancies, and you need to feel comfortable working with him or
her. In the next chapter, we will describe your role in helping
to detect early signs of preterm labor. First, a few words about
your health care providers.

We recommend that your prenatal care be closely supervised by an obstetrician. Although a midwife or general practitioner may be fine for low-risk pregnancies—and could be
fine for your pregnancy as well—an obstetrician brings training and experience in managing more complicated cases. If

you require medication or other treatment, you must be seeing an obstetrician. (Some women with high-risk pregnancies have worked successfully with a midwife in settings where an obstetrician is easily and quickly available in case problems do arise.)

The Obstetrician

You may be seeking a private doctor or be with a hospital clinic or a Health Maintenance Organization (such as the Kaiser system in California). Clearly, the extent of choice available to you will differ. In many clinics or prepaid plans, however, there is some choice among several individual physicians.

It is often difficult to know where to begin when choosing a physician. Ask your family physician for recommendations or call your local hospital maternity unit for names of physicians. Friends may not always know of providers with experience in high-risk pregnancy, but friends are one source of names. Obtain names of several physicians and arrange to meet with each of them. It is perfectly reasonable and important to interview each physician with prepared questions addressing your individual situation and concerns about your pregnancy.

Following are several questions to help you in this process, whether you are choosing a private doctor in your community, selecting among physicians in a group, or just getting to know your chosen provider. You should be able to arrange for a "talking only" appointment to discuss questions with the doctor. There are no right answers to these questions; rather, they are suggested as keys to finding out more about the provider, how helpful she or he is at answering your concerns, and what his or her practices and philosophies are. All of the topics mentioned in these questions are covered in later chapters of this book.

1. What proportion of pregnant women in his or her practice have been high risk? (Your provider should either have experience managing high-risk pregnancies or should already have an arrangement for consultation with a high-risk specialist when needed. You may wish to speak with this specialist, too.)

2. How often will you have prenatal visits? Who will you actually see—are there partners involved in your care? Will one person be the primary provider?

3. Will you have any restrictions on your activity prior to the onset of labor? (See whether you and the doctor can work out the best plan for your situation.)

4. Will she or he help you learn to monitor your own uterine activity? How will you report on your monitoring? Whom can you call if you suspect early signs of preterm labor? What will happen next?

5. How does she or he treat preterm labor? What methods of diagnosis and treatment are most frequently used?

6. What would be the first step if signs of preterm labor are detected? Then what?

7. What kinds of cases does he or she not treat—that is, when is a preterm delivery allowed to occur?

8. What if you feel uncertain or disagree with his or her recommendation?

9. If bedrest seems helpful in your case, will home visits be possible?

10. Where will you deliver if you do have a preterm birth? Will a pediatrician be present at the delivery? Does the hospital have an intensive care nursery?

Things to consider after talking with the physician:

- **Do you feel comfortable talking to this person—especially asking questions?**

- **Does she or he answer questions adequately?**

- **Does her or his philosophy regarding childbirth and medical intervention agree with yours?**

- **Do you agree with his or her management of preterm labor?**

- **Do you think you will be able to participate as you want in the decision-making process?**

- **Do you feel comfortable about any colleagues or other practitioners involved in your care** (such as other physicians or a nurse practioner)?

If your answer to any of these questions is "No," explore the possibilities of finding another obstetrician.

The Pediatrician

Many people wait until the last moment, or until their baby is born, to choose a pediatrician. For women who are at risk for preterm labor, we think it is a good idea to select a pediatrician early. That way, you can feel reassured that if you deliver sooner than you thought, your baby will be in good hands. Your pediatrician can be involved in your baby's care from the start, and get to know your child's individual needs. Again, you may wish to speak with several pediatricians. Here are some questions to include:

1. Does he or she have experience caring for a premature infant in the hospital? After the infant is discharged from the hospital? (Most premature infants are cared for by hospital pediatricians who specialize in newborn infant care, called *neonatologists—see Chapter Nine.* They will be happy to consult with your pediatrician about your baby's progress. If your baby is born early, you may want to choose a pediatrician who has experience caring for prematurely born infants *after* they have gone home.)

2. Will he or she consult with neonatologists while the baby is in the hospital?

3. As the baby gets older, how involved are the parents in making decisions about health care for the baby?

In addition, notice questions the pediatrician asks you; they can give you an idea of the pediatrician's emphasis and style in working with parents. Again, you want to choose a physician with whom you can discuss your concerns. Do you feel comfortable asking questions? Are the answers adequate? Take some time to decide in choosing a pediatrician, but do not wait until labor (whether preterm or not) begins.

One final suggestion: Be wary of providers or hospitals that seem to employ "blanket procedures"—that is, treatment procedures that are the same for everyone—rather than following individual cases and treating according to indicated needs, whether during pregnancy, during labor, at the time of delivery, or after your child is born.

3

Self-
Monitoring
for Preterm
Labor

After the first 20 weeks of pregnancy, one of your most important activities is to feel your uterus for unusual contractions or " tightening."* Early recognition of excessive uterine tightening and other early signs of preterm labor can be a key to preventing preterm birth. The two main questions when monitoring for preterm labor are:

1. Are you noticing a *change* from what has been normal for you?

2. Are you experiencing uterine activity that may be preterm labor?

This book should help you differentiate normal contractions from contractions that may indicate preterm labor.

*You may wish to start monitoring prior to 20 weeks. However, it is questionable whether treatment of uterine activity is effective or desirable before 20 weeks' gestation.

Since one goal is to detect your individual changes, it is important for you to become familiar first with what is normal for you. Once you learn how to monitor for uterine activity, you will need to practice several times each day. Keeping a record will help you learn your own patterns. You will also notice that doing certain activities causes you to have a few contractions. As you gain experience, you may be able to modify your daily routine to avoid activities that do cause contractions.

Remember, every woman and every pregnancy are different. It is normal to have occasional contractions during pregnancy. You are in a key position to identify subtle changes in the way you feel and the frequency of uterine activity you are having. By taking time out each day to monitor for uterine tightenings, you can feel confident about noticing these changes and alerting your prenatal care provider. Developing this daily habit of self-monitoring can mean that you are capable of detecting preterm labor before it reaches advanced stages. This may prevent your baby from being born too early.

What are the Signs and Symptoms of Preterm Labor?

Many of the early warning signs of preterm labor are subtle and develop slowly. Many "symptoms," including contractions, are present during a normal pregnancy. You may not always be able to identify a specific problem; you may just feel that something is different from what you have previously experienced. As you read the list of signs and symptoms below, the question to keep in mind is whether a change has appeared from what has been normal for you.

1. Contractions: A contraction is the tightening of the uterine muscle. The type of contractions that you feel in preterm labor may be different from those felt in term labor. There is usually *no pain* with early preterm labor. You may feel only a tightening of the muscle. Sometimes, you may feel the contraction only if you have your fingers on the uterus to feel for the tightening. Occasionally, you may see the uterus tighten and appear to rise up like a ball.

In this chapter, we describe the procedure for monitoring uterine activity. Again, it is normal to have contractions during pregnancy, but you need to watch for an *increase in frequency or contractions that come at regular intervals*. You should not have four or more contractions or tightenings in one hour, *or* contractions should not be less than 15 minutes apart while you are lying down. If you have *fewer* than four contractions per hour, this uterine activity is probably normal and needs only your careful observation.

2. Menstrual-like cramps: You may feel cramps in the lower part of your abdomen. These are often felt as dull, aching cramps just above the pubic bone. They may be continuous or come and go in a rhythmic pattern.

3. Low backache: Backache is very common during pregnancy, especially as your baby grows. The backache you experience in preterm labor is usually located in the lower back. It may come in waves and may travel to the front of your abdomen. This ache is not relieved by changing your position. It may also come and go, and seem different from the normal backache you have felt at other times during your pregnancy.

4. Abdominal cramps: Abdominal or intestinal cramps, with or without diarrhea, can be associated with preterm labor. Even if you know that you have the flu, persistent diarrhea may cause irritation of the uterus, which can lead to excessive uterine contractions.

5. Pelvic pressure: Women sometimes describe this pressure as a feeling that the baby will "fall out." You may feel you need to move your bowels, but with no result. This feeling of pressure may be constant or may come and go. You also may need to urinate more frequently.

6. Increase or change in vaginal discharge: Many women have increased vaginal discharge during pregnancy. However, any of the following *changes* may be a sign of preterm labor:

- **change in *type* of discharge**

- **increased** *amount* **of discharge**

- **change in** *consistency* **or feel**

- **change in** *color,* **especially to a brown or pink**

If you see a vaginal discharge or have any other symptoms that are different from what is normal for you, notify your physician.

How to Monitor

Monitoring your own uterine activity means lying down and feeling your uterus carefully with your fingertips. We have outlined the method below. We encourage you to ask your health care provider to work with you in practicing these steps until you have learned "the feel" of your own uterus and its contractions.

It is essential to practice monitoring yourself each day. In this way, you can become familiar with your normal pattern of uterine activity. In addition, you may occasionally have contractions that you will not be aware of unless you have your hands on your uterus.

1. When monitoring, lie down, tilting toward your left side. You may put a small pillow under your hip to support your back.*

2. Using your fingertips, gently feel the uterus for tightening (*see figure 6*). Think of your uterus as divided into four sections, and feel over each of the four sections. When the uterus is relaxed, you will be able to indent it with your fingers. During a contraction, the uterus will feel firm to the touch. You will notice a definite pressure change. If you are having a contraction, the entire uterine muscle will become firm.

Sometimes you may feel the baby move. The uterus may feel firm on one side while the opposite side remains soft. You may also have localized contractions that cause a bulging on only one side of the uterus. This type of contraction does not

---

*You should not lie flat on your back during pregnancy for two reasons. First, as the uterus grows, the weight of the baby puts pressure on the *vena cava*, a large vein that flows underneath the baby. This may cause the circulation to you and the baby to decrease. Second, lying on your back may cause you to have more uterine contractions.

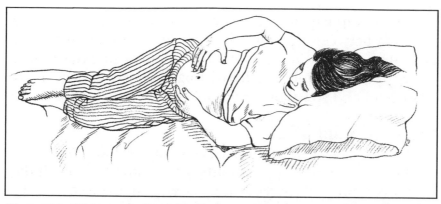

Figure 6 — Using your fingertips, indent your uterus over the entire surface to feel the firmness of the muscle. When your uterus is relaxed, your abdomen will indent easily.

cause equal pressure within the uterus and does not cause your cervix to change. You are monitoring especially to detect contractions that feel uniformly firm over all four sections of your uterus.

3. If you feel uterine tightenings, try to determine how often they are coming and how long they last. When timing these contractions, start counting minutes from the time the uterus begins to tighten. The time from the beginning of a tightening until the uterus becomes soft again is the *length*, or *duration*, of a single contraction. The number of contractions in any given time period (for example, one hour) is the *frequency* of contractions (*see figure 7.*)

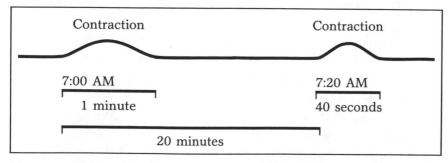

Figure 7 — This example shows that at 7:00 a.m. your uterus tightens, remains firm for one minute, and then relaxes. The next contraction begins at 7:20 a.m. and your uterus remains firm for 40 seconds, then relaxes. The interval between these two contractions is 20 minutes. The first contraction lasted one minute and the second contraction lasted 40 seconds.

4. If you have four or more contractions in an hour, or the time between the beginning of one contraction and the beginning of the next is less than 15 minutes, and this uterine activity persists while you are resting, then you may be in preterm labor and you should contact your health care provider.

When to Monitor

Twice a day, lie down for half an hour and monitor for contractions. Do this at approximately the same time each day, whenever most of your uterine activity seems to occur. For example, certain women feel that their uterus is most active in the afternoon or at night. Others sense more activity in the morning. Whichever is true for you is the time to monitor yourself.

In addition to these regular times, you may notice what seems to be an increase in contractions at some other time of day. At those times, monitor for an hour to check for increased uterine activity. Another important time to monitor is following physical activity, such as swimming, walking a distance, after intercourse or orgasm, or when doing chores. Even if you do not notice contractions, you could be having contractions that you cannot feel until you monitor yourself. Finally, if any of the other signs of preterm labor occur, monitor for contractions when you first notice the sign, and more often thereafter.

A rule of thumb: If any signs or symptoms appear, or if in doubt, *monitor for contractions.*

A pregnant woman speaks:

There were times when I found myself resisting feeling my uterus after I had noticed a possible increase of contractions. I just didn't want to find out that I was, in fact, having too many contractions—I was worried about what that would mean. I got over that resistance quickly by remembering the baby we lost because preterm labor was not detected early enough to stop it. During that pregnancy, I did not know I was "high risk," nor did I learn what early contractions feel like. This time, I was determined to help catch any problems early. So, I just forced myself to monitor whenever there might be a need, even if I wanted, for a moment, to deny it.

Keep a Daily Record

It will be very helpful if you write down, each day, any uterine contractions, as well as the activity you were engaged in at the time. The sample "Daily Log" worksheet (*see figure 8*) provides a useful format for recording your contractions and what you were doing at the time. Use it to keep track of your regular monitoring sessions, as well as any other times you feel contractions or other preterm labor signs.

When documenting your contractions during monitoring sessions or other times, write down the time each contraction starts and the length of each contraction. Check (✓) if you are having any other signs of labor. You may notice that you experience one of these signs, but you do not have any contractions. This is reassuring, but continue to watch for uterine activity. Write down what you were doing at the time you began to monitor or when you noticed you were having contractions. This may help you determine what types of activities cause you to have contractions; if you can modify your activity, you may have fewer uterine contractions. Once you and your doctor become familiar with your normal pattern (for example, you usually have one or two contractions per hour), you can concentrate on marking down any changes in frequency, duration, or how strong they feel.

It is also interesting to note whether your mood seems to affect your uterine activity. Write down a description of your mood when you are monitoring. You may find you have more contractions at times you feel a bit low and fewer contractions when your mood is better. We do not know which may be cause and which effect. However, if it is possible to alter your situation in ways that might help your mood (and this is not always possible), give it a try. (Note: The bottom section on the Daily Log is for recording medications you may be taking to slow contractions, and your pulse just before taking the drug, and again 30 to 40 minutes after. For discussion of these medications, and instructions on pulse-taking, *see Chapter Seven.*)

Questions Often Asked about Uterine Monitoring:

Q. *I've heard of contractions called "Braxton-Hicks" that*

Preterm Labor Monitoring Worksheet

Name _____ Phone _____ Doctor _____ Due Date _____

	Date	Time	Date	Time	Date	Time	Date	Time
Contractions:								
Interval between? (min.)								
How long? (sec.)								
Do you feel:								
Tightening								
Cramps								
Pressure								
Low Backache								
Intestinal cramps or diarrhea								
Increase or change in vaginal discharge								
Activity What are you doing when contractions occur?								
Mood Scale 1–4 1 = depressed or discouraged 4 = happy, everything is great								
Medications Pulse rate								

Figure 8 — Daily Log.

nearly all pregnant women seem to have. What are these, and how will I know if I am having them?

A. Braxton-Hicks contractions are painless tightenings that occur normally during pregnancy. They often feel similar to preterm labor contractions, and there is no sure way to distinguish between the two kinds of uterine activity. Braxton-Hicks contractions do not usually come in a definite pattern, their frequency is almost always less than one contraction per hour, and they do *not* cause your cervix to change. It is important, however, not to ignore contractions by saying "Oh, they are only Braxton-Hicks." It is also important not to rely on a friend, sister, mother, aunt, pregnancy book, nurse, or doctor who may tell you the same thing. Again, monitor for *frequency* and *duration*, as described earlier.

Remember, contractions that occur with preterm labor are also usually painless. They begin slowly, and may hardly be noticeable. In other words, you cannot consider *pain* as a sign of preterm labor. Pain often appears very late in labor. By the time pain is present, preterm labor may be too far advanced for effective treatment to stop it.

From this time on, do not even consider the word *pain* as an important characteristic of preterm labor contractions.

Q. *Can my partner or a friend help me with my daily uterine monitoring?*

A. Good idea! An important part of monitoring may be the help and support you receive from your partner or a friend. He or she can help you identify contractions and time them. There may be times you do not want to believe you are actually having contractions, and it may be important to have another person say, "Yes, these are contractions and they are regular." Your partner or friend can practice feeling for uterine tightening by placing his or her hands on your uterus and gently feeling each of the four sections, just the way you do. See if you both agree about what a contraction feels like. In our experience, the partner frequently identifies contractions before the mother-to-be recognizes them. In some cases, the partner's monitoring has been helpful in detecting preterm labor and getting to the hospital in time.

If you are a single woman or your partner is not available during the times you monitor each day (or your partner is just not the person to do this with you, for whatever reason), a friend or family member may be able to work out a daily routine with you. Whoever does monitor with you can also be a great emotional support. It is not easy for some women to lie down and monitor their uterus twice a day, especially if they are used to being active and independent. Encouragement from someone else can make this task much easier. Try to turn daily monitoring, and keeping a Daily Log, into an activity that is not so bad after all, an activity that can keep you going because you know you are on top of things and taking good care of yourself and your baby.

Q. *How will I know that I'm monitoring correctly?*

A. When you are first learning to monitor, practice with your physician or nurse. Take your Daily Log to your regular prenatal visits, go over it with your provider, and double-check on the way you feel your uterus. Talk over with your provider any activities you do that seem to be associated with increased uterine tightenings. Perhaps you can change these activities in some way until after your baby is born.

What to Do if You Detect Frequent or Regular Uterine Tightening

The purpose of daily monitoring is to catch early signs that may indicate preterm labor is occurring. Becoming familiar with steps you would follow if you do think you are experiencing regular or frequent uterine tightening can let you feel more comfortable throughout your pregnancy, knowing that potential problems will be handled appropriately.

1. If you have detected regular, frequent contractions for one hour or more while lying down, call your physician and tell him or her your name, the number of weeks since your last menstrual period, and your particular risk factor for preterm delivery, if you know it (*see the list of conditions in Chapter One*).

2. Tell your physician whether or not you are taking medication to decrease uterine contractions. If you are, give the dosage, the time you last took the medication, and your pulse rate.

3. Report how often your contractions are coming or how many you have had in the last hour.

4. Report how active you have been during the day, what you had been doing before noticing contractions. (You should be lying down while monitoring, but what were you doing before that?)

5. Describe any other signs of labor you may be experiencing.

If for any reason you are unable to speak directly with your physician within 30 minutes, or if you reach a doctor or nurse who tells you to "Wait and see what happens," we suggest you "play it safe" instead: Go to the labor and delivery unit in your hospital. The nurse can call your physician after you arrive. There, you will be monitored for uterine contractions and have your cervix examined to determine if you *are* in preterm labor. If you are not, you can feel reassured that everything is fine, and you can return home.

Most of us are not used to making this kind of decision in a medical situation, perhaps against a doctor or nurse's advice. However, it is very important *not* to be concerned or feel silly about going "unnecessarily" to the hospital. The worst thing that can happen if you *do* go to the hospital but are not in preterm labor is that you may feel you have gone for nothing. This is not true. It is both helpful and reassuring to know that your cervix has not dilated. If you *do not* go, you run the risk of a much worse outcome—delivering a premature baby.

When Should You Act? A Doctor's View:

Quite often, patients feel embarrassed about waking their practitioner up in the middle of the night. You should realize, however, that your practitioner can probably catch up on his or her sleep the next day. But if your baby is born preterm, there is nothing that can place him or her back in your womb the next day!

As a matter of fact, when our preterm birth prevention program was started, there was a concern that over-anxious patients would make many unnecessary visits and calls to the labor and delivery unit. To our great surprise, this did not happen. Only very rarely does a mother-to-be feel that something is wrong with her uterine activity when nothing is happening. In most of the cases, the visits or calls have been necessary.

When Should You Act? A Pregnant Woman's View:

This book provides guidelines about what to do and when to do it. But I still may not always feel completely clear about it. When I monitor contractions, I am not always absolutely sure if I feel one—a mild contraction is not always obvious. Or, if I'm trying to keep track of contractions unobtrusively (say in the middle of a work meeting, or when friends are over for dinner), I may not be totally sure how many contractions I've had in an hour. Or, even if I'm pretty sure I've had six or eight contractions in an hour, I don't always feel confident that they are serious enough to warrant lying down or calling the doctor.

In these circumstances, I've decided to follow this book's advice—to play it safe and be cautious. I've decided it is far, far better to be wrong a hundred times by being too careful than to be wrong once by ignoring signs of impending preterm labor. The biggest obstacle to acting is likely to be embarrassment. It is embarrassing to leave a meeting or a dinner because I think I'm having contractions; it is embarrassing to call the doctor and be told it's 'false labor,' or 'Braxton-Hicks.' However, in this case the alternative is too important to let this affect my actions.

CHAPTER

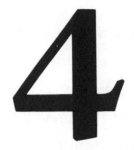

The
Diagnosis of
Preterm
Labor

Your own daily monitoring for excessive uterine activity and for other possible signs of preterm labor is one important aspect of detecting preterm labor (*see Chapter Three*). The second is the actual *diagnosis*, by an experienced obstetrician, who will determine whether you are in early stages of preterm labor. You do not want to be treated for preterm labor if you are not having preterm labor.

Before describing how this diagnosis is made, here is a quick review of what "labor" is (*see Chapter One*). Labor means that two events are occurring at the same time:

1. Regular contractions of the uterine muscle are present (the often misleading expression "labor pains"—remember, these contractions may be painless); and

2. The cervix (opening of the uterus, or womb, into the

vagina) changes. These changes, which can be discovered through a pelvic examination by a health professional, include:

- **opening of the cervix** (*dilation*) (*see figure 9*)

- **shortening of the cervix** (*effacement*) (*see figure 9*)

- **softening of the cervix**

- **altered position of the cervix**

- **descent of the baby into the pelvis** (*entry*; sometimes called *dropping*) (*see figure 10*)

The maintenance of pregnancy is a delicate balance between two forces: One force tries to push the baby out (the uterine contractions); the other works to keep the baby inside (the resistance of the uterine cervix). When the balance between uterine contractions and cervical resistance remains normal, the pregnancy is expected to go full term. A disturbance in the balance prior to 37 weeks of pregnancy may result in preterm labor. Too many uterine contractions* too early in pregnancy may upset the balance and cause cervical changes, followed by preterm delivery. Or, in some cases, cervical changes may occur without excessive uterine activity because of a "weakness" of the uterine cervix—that is, the cervix does not provide adequate resistance to the weight of the fetus and/or to minimal uterine activity. This condition is often called cervical incompetence. (For further discussion, *see Chapter Six*.)

It is often difficult to distinguish which comes first—uterine activity or cervical changes. If you or your health care provider suspect signs of preterm labor, however, the diagnostic process will include checking for each.

Checking Uterine Activity

In Chapter Three, we described how you can monitor your own uterine activity by feeling with your fingertips and keeping a daily record. This type of monitoring is considered

---

*Keep in mind that one pregnant woman's "normal balance" is likely to differ from another's; the same number and/or strength of contractions may cause cervical changes for one woman but not for the other, depending on how much resistance each cervix provides.

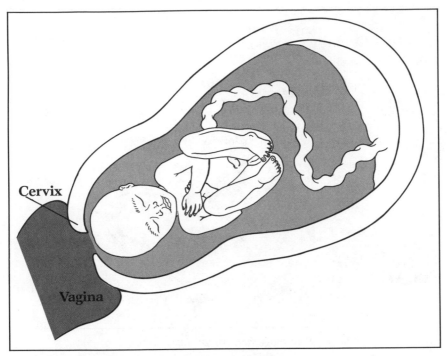

Figure 9 — Cervix thinning (effacing) and dilating.

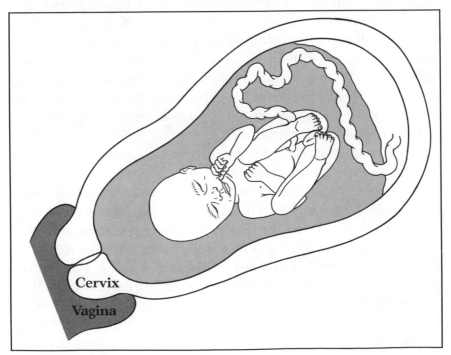

Figure 10 — Descent of the baby into the pelvis.

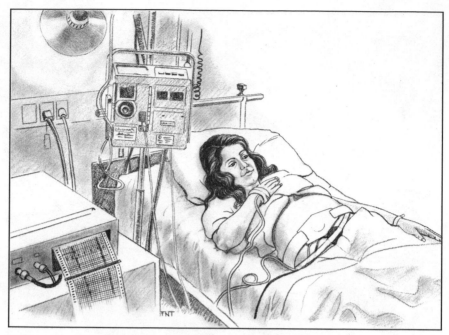

Figure 11 — In-hospital management of preterm labor.

"subjective," as it is based on your own interpretations. The advantage of this method is that it can be done at any time and any place, with minimal expense. However, with this method, you may not detect all your uterine contractions, particularly when the uterine wall is very tense—for example, in twin or triplet pregnancies. Also, intestinal cramps, a full bladder, or fetal movements may occasionally give you the false sensation of contractions.

The second method for monitoring uterine activity uses an instrument that measures and records uterine contractions. If you or your practitioner suspect excessive contractions based upon feeling your uterus, a monitoring instrument will be used to obtain an "objective" measure. Monitoring instruments that record uterine activity and fetal heart rate are now available in all hospitals and in some practitioners' offices. These monitors are probably more reliable in detecting contractions than self-monitoring. However, instrument monitors have the obvious disadvantage of limiting your freedom to move around (*see figure 11*). If instrument monitoring over a long time period is desired, you must be in a hospital, unless your doctor

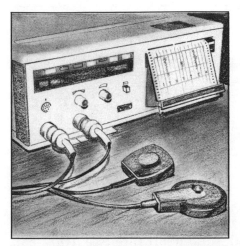

Figure 12 — Monitor with transducers to record uterine contractions and fetal heart rate.

considers it safe to monitor at home.* Since instruments are not perfect, they should be double-checked if you feel contractions that do not appear on the monitor. Also, it is probably advisable to check periodically for cervical changes even during instrumental monitoring.

A monitor for uterine contractions and fetal heart rate is shown in *figure 12.*

One of the transducers uses *ultrasound,* or soundwaves, to measure the fetus's heart rate. This transducer is placed on your abdomen at the location where the fetal heart can best be heard. In order to improve the sound quality, a special gel is applied to your skin. Women frequently ask about the safety of ultrasound for a fetus. Ultrasound has been used for years without evidence of harmful effects. Nevertheless, to be on the safe side, the ultrasound fetal heart rate monitoring function of the machinery can be turned off while uterine contraction monitoring continues. Ask your practitioner to use the ultrasound transducer only when a measure of the fetal heart rate is needed.

The other transducer (called tocodynamometer) is usually placed on top of your uterus and kept on the skin with a snug belt. This part of the monitor uses no ultrasound. It measures changes in pressure caused by contractions. Occasionally, fetal kicks or coughing and sneezing by you may be picked up too, but they produce different patterns on the monitor strip.

The transducers do not cause significant discomfort while in use. As the monitoring is done, a strip of recording paper

*Recently, a portable monitor has been developed that allows a woman to measure uterine contractions at home and transmit the information, through the telephone, to trained nurses and the woman's doctor. The woman need not remain in the hospital just to be monitored. As with any medical device or procedure, the value of home uterine monitors must be established through well-designed studies. Early studies are promising, indicating that home monitoring can help identify excessive contractions and contribute to treatment decisions. (*See figure 23, page 104.*)

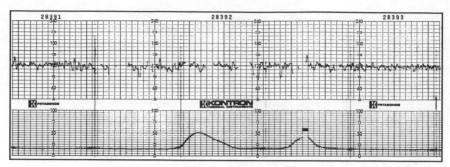

Figure 13 — Sample monitor record. Top: Fetal heart rate. Bottom: Uterine contractions.

rolls out of the monitoring box, showing the pattern of your uterine activity and, if desired, fetal heart rate (*see figure 13*).

When using an instrument to monitor uterine contractions your practitioner considers the same basic characteristics that you do in self-monitoring:

1. Regularity: What is the time interval between each contraction? If roughly the same each time, such as every five or 10 minutes, the contractions are considered regular. If the interval between contractions varies, they are considered irregular. Irregular contractions are less likely to produce cervical changes.

2. Frequency: How often do the contractions occur? In general, the more often the contractions occur, the more likely they are to result in cervical changes.

3. Duration: How long does each contraction last? Contractions may last only a few seconds, or as long as a minute or even two minutes. The longer they last, the more likely they are to represent contractions of labor.

4. Intensity: How strong are the contractions? The strength of a contraction is generally reflected in how tight the abdomen feels, but is not related to whether pain is felt. Stronger contractions produce higher pressure in the uterus, and are more likely to represent real labor.

Checking Cervical Change
The second aspect of the diagnostic process focuses on the other factor defining "labor": changes in the cervix. If either

self-monitoring or instrument-monitoring indicates possible excessive uterine activity, a pelvic examination is performed to see whether cervical changes, as described earlier, are occurring.

We usually recommend a woman be observed for a while in the hospital for both uterine activity and cervical changes (as checked by a pelvic exam). If instrument-monitoring shows regular uterine contractions, and if they are accompanied by changes in the cervix, the diagnosis of preterm labor is made. If uterine activity is *not* accompanied by changes in the cervix, however, monitoring is usually continued until this activity returns to normal or until a change in the cervix is detected by a later pelvic examination. In the absence of cervical change, the woman can return home, especially if she keeps careful watch over her uterine activity and is able to come back for instrument monitoring, if necessary. In other words, as long as no cervical changes can be detected, medical treatment is probably not required. Repeated uterine monitoring (self and instrument) is a good idea, especially in cases where the diagnosis is not clear. On the other hand, if cervical changes do appear, different steps will need to be taken (*see figure 14*).

If the Diagnosis of Preterm Labor Is Made

At the present time, no single method has been identified as the most successful in stopping preterm labor. However, most practitioners follow the steps outlined below when managing a patient with early signs of preterm labor or with persistent, excessive uterine activity:

Step 1. Bedrest (*see Chapter Five*) and continued monitoring of uterine activity; repeat pelvic examination to check for cervical changes. If no improvement . . .

Step 2-A. Search for treatable cause of excessive uterine activity, such as urinary tract infection, intestinal infection (diarrhea), etc., through laboratory studies (urine test, cervical culture for bacteria), and physical exam (taking temperature and pulse, listening to lungs, etc.).

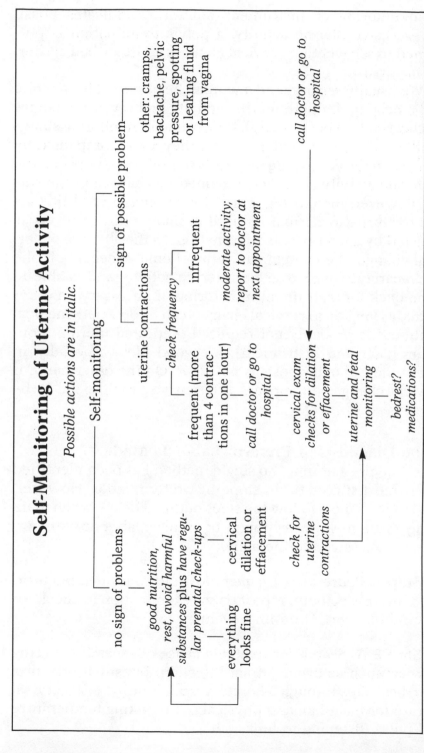

Self-Monitoring of Uterine Activity

Possible actions are in italic.

Self-monitoring

no sign of problems

good nutrition, rest, avoid harmful substances plus have regular prenatal check-ups

everything looks fine

cervical dilation or effacement

check for uterine contractions

uterine and fetal monitoring

bedrest? medications?

cervical exam checks for dilation or effacement

sign of possible problem

uterine contractions

check frequency

frequent (more than 4 contractions in one hour)

call doctor or go to hospital

infrequent

moderate activity; report to doctor at next appointment

other: cramps, backache, pelvic pressure, spotting or leaking fluid from vagina

call doctor or go to hospital

Figure 14 — Possible events during pregnancy. Remember, every case must be treated on an individual basis, with close cooperation between you and your health care providers.

Step 2-B. In some cases, intravenous fluids (hydration) and/or medication to ease restlessness or anxiety (sedation) are used, in the belief that dehydration and/or anxiety may increase uterine activity.*

Step 3. If signs of preterm labor continue to develop after the above procedures have been followed, a more aggressive intervention may be necessary. In most cases, medications will be given that can stop uterine contractions (called *tocolytic* medications). For discussion of these medications, *see Chapter Eight.*

How Certain Is a Diagnosis of Preterm Labor?

In diagnosing and treating preterm labor, as in other areas of health care, answers cannot always be certain. Physicians cannot always be *sure* if a woman is in preterm labor, particularly in its early stages. The questions of when to consider the woman in need of treatment, and what type of intervention to use, require weighing the risks and benefits of the available options, a process best done cooperatively by an experienced practitioner and an informed patient.

When trying to detect preterm labor early enough to treat it effectively, medical providers may give medication or other treatment to some women who would have done just fine and continued to full term without any medical intervention other than bedrest and continued monitoring. However, waiting in every case for very strong contractions and advanced cervical changes before starting treatment could mean that some of the treatments will be much less effective than if they had been started earlier. Delayed treatment, therefore, may not be as effective overall in preventing preterm births.

We would all prefer certainty when diagnosing and treating a health condition. In the case of preterm labor, it is especially important for a high-risk woman to understand the possible trade-offs of treatment versus waiting, and give some thought to what she would want to do *before* a problem

*The decision to give fluids must be made with care. If a woman must be given medication to stop contractions soon after this hydration procedure, the increased fluid may cause unwanted side effects (*see Chapter 8*). With regard to sedation (morphine or a barbiturate), no long-term effects on the fetus are known, although it is "made sleepy" temporarily by this sedation. If a preterm birth does occur within the next couple of hours, the newborn may receive an "antidote" to the medication.

actually develops. Because babies born very prematurely can face a number of serious health problems, it seems acceptable to risk a limited amount of over-diagnosis and treatment of early signs of preterm labor to try to avoid a very preterm delivery. In other words, the known risks of treatment to stop preterm labor, when supervised by an experienced obstetric staff, are much less than the tremendous health risks for a very premature infant.

As a well-informed obstetric patient, you can and should be involved in decisions about diagnosis and treatment of preterm labor if troublesome signs do appear. Sometimes, women who monitor themselves carefully and report to their practitioner's office or to the labor unit with excessive uterine activity will be sent home because no cervical changes can be found during pelvic examination. However, you *must not* get discouraged about self-monitoring or embarrassed about coming back again and again if uterine activity again becomes excessive. We encourage repeated monitoring by instrument, as well as pelvic exams when necessary in questionable cases. (In some cases, cervical exams should be limited or even avoided completely, such as when there is placenta previa or ruptured membranes.) The fact that uterine activity did not cause changes in the cervix one time does *not* guarantee that cervical changes will not be present in the future. On the contrary, it is not unusual for a woman to detect excessive uterine activity before her physician can detect cervical changes. Only when the woman insists on returning to be examined can cervical changes ultimately be detected and appropriate treatment started.

Remember, in order to avoid overtreatment, we do want to wait for *both* uterine activity and cervical changes. However, if you detect excessive uterine activity after being sent home once or twice without any detectable cervical changes, don't assume the next time will be the same. If you return to the hospital and everything is fine, nothing is lost. But if you *don't* return, and preterm labor advances, premature delivery may result! Don't worry that you may be reacting to a "false alarm." It is not "false" if you detect excessive uterine activity. Like the fire department, we'd rather check on suspicions of smoke than wait to see definite flames. In fact, our experience has shown that high-risk women who are educated about early signs of preterm labor become very good judges of their own condition. With most of our program participants, the pregnant mother-to-be is correct in her perception of excessive uterine activity.

In summary, if you have doubts about whether you may be experiencing preterm labor, contact your health care provider. *Do not* hesitate. Everyone will feel better if your *early diagnosis* prevents *early delivery*.

CHAPTER

5

Bedrest

at

Home

During pregnancy, many women try to spend some extra time resting in bed—taking afternoon naps, "sleeping late" in the morning. For some women, however, staying in bed becomes a prescribed activity during a portion of their pregnancy. Your obstetrician may prescribe bedrest for one of two general reasons:

1. You have had symptoms that might develop into preterm labor, but do not require more aggressive intervention, such as medications or cerclage (*described in Chapters Six and Seven*). For example, if monitoring, by you or monitoring instrument, shows excessive uterine activity but a pelvic exam shows no cervical changes, your doctor may send you home "on bedrest."

2. You are diagnosed as having preterm labor that can be treated by medications or cerclage. Treatment begins in the hospital, followed by bedrest at home along with oral medications to stop uterine contractions.

There are differing degrees of bedrest. Women on *complete bedrest* should not get out of bed at all, even to use the bathroom. (These women become experienced users of bedpans and sponge baths!) Less restricted bedrest allows you to get up for certain reasons: for bathroom privileges only; to use the bathroom and prepare one meal a day; to spend one hour each morning and evening up and around your house, etc. If you are allowed to get up, try to avoid using your abdominal muscles to do so. (*See figure 15.*)

The length of time on bedrest—days, weeks, months—will vary according to individual circumstances. Also, the type of bedrest may change over time. Depending on how you respond, physically and emotionally, restrictions may decrease or increase.

There is no set formula defining the level of restriction and amount of allowable activity appropriate for any individual woman. The type of bedrest prescribed is probably best worked out cooperatively by you and your physician after considering several questions:

- **What is your physical condition** (especially, uterine activity and cervical status), **and might bedrest help prevent further problems?**

- **Is your pregnancy at a critical time where delivery would be most dangerous for your baby?** (*See Chapter Nine.*)

- **What specific activities or situations are associated with increased uterine contractions** *for you*, **and does bedrest help avoid these activities?** (Your own daily uterine monitoring will help answer this one.)

- **How feasible are various "degrees" of bedrest, given your home situation?** (For example, is someone available to help with household needs, do you have other children who need care, can you manage financially if you are not working and/or need to hire someone to help out?)

- **How well do you adjust to restrictions of bedrest?** (Some women become upset about staying in bed, making matters worse.)

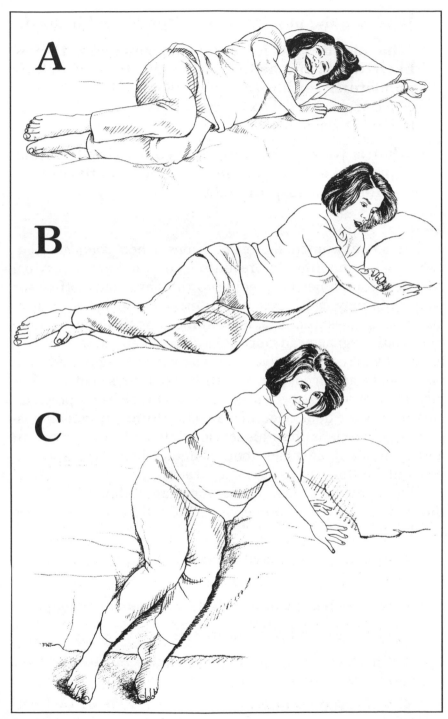

Figure 15 — Getting up from bed. Push on left elbow and hands to avoid using abdominal muscles.

- **What are the physical risks of prolonged bedrest?**

- **What are the risks if you do *not* go on bedrest? How likely would you be to need medication, or deliver prematurely, or stay the same?** (Remember, your physician can provide only an educated guess; there is no way to predict accurately.)

- **What is your evaluation after comparing the risks of preterm delivery to the risks and benefits of bedrest for you and your baby?**

Medical Home Visits

For some women there are times when *complete* bedrest may be important in preventing contractions or cervical changes. Sometimes even going to the physician's office for a checkup may cause excessive uterine activity. Your physician may suggest that your prenatal exams be done at home until your pregnancy advances to a stage when uterine activity is not as worrisome. Or, you can ask your physician if home visits can be arranged. Home visits by your physician, another physician, or nurse experienced in caring for high-risk pregnancies usually are done once a week. Unfortunately, not all hospitals or physicians offer this service. Talk with your physician and local health agencies about whether home visits would be available for you if the need arises.

When you are seen at home, the examination is basically the same as during an office visit. The following procedures can be done:

1. Monitor uterine contractions (by palpation or instrument monitor).

2. Do a pelvic exam to check on cervical changes.

3. Listen to the baby's heart rate.

4. Check your vital signs—temperature, pulse rate, blood pressure.

5. Take urine or blood sample.

6. Check on your weight.

7. Measure the growth of your baby.

There may be benefits to home visits other than saving you the trip and exertion. You have more time to ask questions and discuss concerns about your pregnancy. You may develop a special relationship with your nurse or physician, especially if you are seen over a long period of time.

Feelings: Some Good, Some Bad

Staying in bed requires effort. While sometimes it may sound luxurious to be able to spend more time in bed, *having to stay in bed all the time is difficult for most people*, affecting many areas of their life. Bedrest is more complicated than it may sound. Our aim is to make this experience a little easier, in case you do spend time on bedrest, by sharing with you the reactions and coping strategies of women who have already done it. Keep in mind that everyone's experiences and reactions are individual.

If you find yourself confined to bed during part of your pregnancy, remember that feeling anxious or upset is a common reaction. Pregnant women on bedrest obviously have legitimate concerns—about how their pregnancy will turn out, about their baby's health and their own condition, about the significant changes in their life and the lives of those around them during the time they spend in bed. Here are some of the feelings women report about prolonged bedrest:

"I felt so helpless, lying there in bed all the time . . ."

> *I called myself a 'human incubator.' Suddenly my role in life was to stay in bed. I had always been a very active person. It was hard to give up the control over my life that I usually had . . . it took me four weeks to adjust.*

> *I had to accept help from others for everything, and learn to ask for help, without being able to do anything for them in return. I got used to things being done differently at home, by my friends and partner. I didn't worry about things being less clean or less organized than I was used to in normal times.*

"The isolation got to me sometimes . . ."

Three or four days might pass when the only person I saw was my husband. When he came home, I couldn't stop talking. I'd watch TV for hours just to see other people doing things, and the telephone became my lifeline to sanity and the outside world. As I gradually became used to this confinement, I realized I had made the best choice for my unborn baby and that this was only temporary. I marked my calender in red on the day I knew I could go back to my activities.

"Sometimes, I felt guilty . . ."

I thought back to activities I had done that might have "caused" me to have problems. I'd think, "If only I hadn't walked those three blocks, or done the laundry, or insisted on going to that meeting. If I'd taken better care of myself, would this have happened?" Of course, I had taken good care of myself—watched my diet, followed my doctor's advice, rested. So maybe it was my attitude. Did I somehow think myself or worry myself into having to go to bed? Or secretly wish I could just relax? All the prenatal books I read just made me feel worse. They said that to have a healthy baby, all you do is eat right, exercise, rest, and see your doctor. Where did I go wrong?

I finally realized that these thoughts were getting me nowhere, and that in most cases no one knows what causes the problems requiring bedrest. I was glad I was now doing what was needed to handle the problem.

"I must have seemed pretty self-centered . . ."

I was concerned about being comfortable, about what I ate, and about not being disturbed. And of course, I wasn't lifting a finger to help with chores. I didn't appear to be sick or suffering to people who visited. Maybe I didn't really need to be on bedrest anyway. No one could say for sure I'd deliver prematurely. What if I was just "pampering" myself?

But pregnancy is a time when many women become preoccupied with themselves. I learned to explain to other people
that I needed to stay off my feet. I wasn't pampering myself,
I was pampering my unborn baby—and rightfully so! Most
important, I learned to trust my own informed decisions about
what was best to do or not do, and to politely ignore well-
intentioned but less-informed advice from friends, aunts, in-
laws, parents, neighbors.

"My self-image really tumbled . . ."

I prided myself on being really healthy and on getting
through my first pregnancy without "missing a beat" in my
work. I got a lot of self-esteem from my work and from my
image of myself as a healthy, productive person. I had envi-
sioned working up until a week before the baby was due. When
I had to go on bedrest I felt as if my body had failed me, and
as if I had failed in my job as a working woman.

Somehow, to be put on bedrest made me feel as if I were
inadequate. And it doesn't help to be in a lying-down position
to everyone around you. It's much harder to be assertive and
confident.

"I realize I was pretty moody . . ."

Sometimes I felt as if I could handle everything with no
trouble, and five minutes later I was sure I'd never last till
term without unraveling. How was I going to stay in bed for
13 weeks? Of course, the truth was in between: I made it,
but at times things felt pretty rocky. In the beginning, the
slightest thing said to me might make me cry, especially from
my husband. Here I was, feeling trapped, having to ask for
every bite of food or drink, or errands to be done. I had to
become a "pain in the neck," even to the most patient partner. I was worried about all he was having to do on top of
trying to get his usual work done, yet I had no choice about
being so dependent. We were both "trapped" in this situation. At low times, I questioned having this baby—the baby

we both wanted seemed to be causing a strain even on our very strong relationship, rather than being a source of joy and "togetherness." Having those feelings just upset me more.

We just had to keep reminding ourselves that this situation was temporary, by no means our usual or permanent state. The goal was still the baby, who would become a permanent addition to the family and the life we had before.

"I worried about work I should be doing . . ."

Even though I was supposed to take it easy, I had visions of efficient women using their time in bed to write novels or reports, or at least to catch up on correspondence. I felt guilty that my partner had to take on so much housework and run all the errands. Much of the time I felt groggy and unfocused and then felt bad that I wasn't doing more.

In my profession there is heavy pressure to keep working against all adversity. I hadn't missed a day of work because of sickness for five years, and now I was supposed to spend five months in bed, when I felt perfectly well. And then how could I think about taking more time off when the baby was born?

Now I couldn't even use my time productively. My ability to concentrate seemed completely gone, and I had no motivation to undertake anything either challenging or even the least boring like that pile of professional literature I'd been putting off reading. I realize in retrospect that those are common and normal responses to being under such stress, but at the time I was embarrased and discouraged. All I wanted to do was distract myself from worrying about what might happen. When I finally accepted that I wasn't going to accomplish a lot, and let myself read magazines and watch TV, I felt much better.

"I just wasn't prepared for this . . ."

Even though I knew I was "high risk," I thought it wouldn't happen to me. So it was a huge mental adjustment, as well as physical, when I found myself on bedrest. It's probably even more of a shock if you are not considered "high risk." Next time, I'd really prepare myself ahead for the possibility of weeks in bed, I'd assume that is likely, and then be pleasantly surprised, and very happy, if it is not necessary.

"And then there were funny times . . ."

Like the sharp pain in my left breast, which, when I finally investigated, turned out to be a large crumb of French bread that had not quite reached my mouth, but had managed to fall under my shirt, wedging itself upon the left nipple.

"Towards the end I was getting impatient . . ."

After many weeks in bed, I found myself feeling rather ambivalent about the last stretch. I really wanted the bedrest to be over. I was more uncomfortable physically as my uterus grew larger, and I was generally getting restless. But I knew that wishing bedrest, and the pregnancy, to be over still meant our baby would be born a bit too early. I resolved to "hang in" each day. Although our baby was now likely to be healthy, I wanted to increase that likelihood as much as possible. When I was able to slowly begin some activity—getting up for a meal, taking a shower—I knew we were almost there and my spirits definitely picked up.

Feelings such as those expressed above tend to come and go. Everyone agrees that bedrest can be difficult. But when it's over, it is over! And the unanimous conclusion is that the "sacrificed" weeks were worth it.

Women who have been on bedrest report that it does get easier after the first week or two. Those first days require much patience as you get organized about meals, work, bathing, household chores, etc. Once new routines are in place, bedrest becomes less difficult. Give yourself and those around you several weeks to adjust mentally and physically to the new limitations on your activity. And again, don't be surprised if you do experience shifts in your mood—"good days and bad days"—throughout the time spent on bedrest; let yourself have a good cry when needed, then get on with your bedrest activities. As time goes by, and a term delivery comes nearer, the "bad days" will probably become less frequent.

Some general advice: Don't get discouraged by the negative feelings; they are to be expected. But remember the positive, and think to the future, especially to the years ahead with the child for whom you are already caring so well.

You will also feel bedrest physically. Muscles do become weak and are likely to ache a bit. You may feel sore spots from lying on your side, so it's a good idea to change positions now and then. You may be able to do mild "bedbound" exercises to keep some muscle tone, although *any* exercises should first be discussed with your physician.

A few words about the end of bedrest, whether at home or in the hospital. As you approach 37 weeks' gestation, talk to your doctor about gradually introducing some physical activity. If you have spent many weeks in bed, expect to feel weak. Even standing to brush your teeth will feel strange and tiring. After your baby is born, you certainly may be more exhausted than other new mothers. If possible, arrange for help, especially with housework, marketing, meals, laundry. If you have been unable to gather clothing and equipment for the baby—or if you prefer to wait until after the birth—ask a family member or friend to help obtain the immediate necessities.

Keep in mind that most women do regain their physical state quite quickly once they are off bedrest. Muscles return, and before long you are back to where you were before all this began.

Adjusting to bedrest, of course, involves much more than coping with emotional ups and downs or physical aches and pains. There are concrete, practical problems that are of particular concern to women on bedrest. These include managing the household, maintaining outside work commitments, reducing social activities, and if you have children, dealing with raising them from your new "permanent" post in the bedroom—all the while trying to be as comfortable and relaxed as possible. You will need to ask your family, friends, and co-workers for special understanding during this time, and for help with arranging and re-arranging routines, chores, people, objects, and schedules.

The following pages provide some suggestions for handling these common problems.

Getting Organized at Home*

Think about where you can lie down comfortably at home. You may want to have your bed moved or rent a hospital bed so that you can be near a window with an interesting view, or nearer the telephone, bathroom, or kitchen. Think about how to vary your scenery, if possible, perhaps lying on the living room sofa or, in good weather, a chaise lounge or hammock outside.

Get dressed in the morning. Don't stay in your pajamas.

A schedule can make it easier to face the day. Include wake up time, work time, craft projects, activities with your partner and children, TV programs you want to watch, and so on. Do various activities to help break up the day.

Make a grocery checklist of foods, brands, and quantities you usually keep on hand, so that someone can do your shopping. Alternatively, post a list and be sure that someone keeps track of what is needed.

Collect take-out menus and deli price lists from all over your area.

Pack a suitcase for going to the hospital for delivery or other treatment. You may want: slippers and/or warm socks, a robe, hairbrush, toothbrush, headband or hair barrette, lip balm, hand cream, aids for labor (such as music or something to look at), clothes and blanket for baby.

Check what your health insurance covers in the event of complications of delivery (such as cesarean section) or extra care for the newborn (such as an intensive-care nursery for a premature baby).

Keep careful records of everything you buy and your expenses for childcare or domestic help. At tax time, these may be deductible as medical or child and dependent care expenses.

---

*These sections have been adapted from "Bed and Bored" by Susan Schwartz. The original pamphlet is available from Birthways, 3127 Telegraph Ave., Oakland, CA 94609.

Plan how to handle money. It's easy to open accounts and make deposits by mail. Getting cash can be more difficult. The easiest way is a joint account with a spouse, or finding someone who will bring you cash and then take your check for it. Before sending someone to your bank to cash a check on your account, call to ask what identification or other information may be required. Write the purpose of the check in the endorsement on the back of the check; for example, "For cash for (your name)." Don't give anyone a blank check, your credit card, or your cash machine card and its code.

Help Around the House

Ask for help no matter how independent you have been. Trying to "go it alone" will leave you too isolated and may force you to do things that endanger your baby. There are people and organizations who will support you: family, friends, fellow employees, churches, charities, government organizations.

List your daily activities and work out who might help with meal preparation, shopping, cleaning, laundry, and helping you get to your doctor or other appointments. A county health department nurse can help with this organizing (*see "Counseling, Information, and Referral," page 73*). Spread out the burdens as much as possible. When friends ask, "Is there anything I can do?" take them up on it with a specific request. If people want to visit, invite them to dinner, but ask them to bring the meal. *Don't* accept your spouse or partner's offer to do it all— few people can work and also take care of a house, a woman confined to bed, and perhaps children.

Hire housekeeping help if you can afford it (financial aid is almost nonexistent). Firms listed in the yellow pages under "Health Care," "Nursing," or "House Cleaning" can supply help quickly and find replacements if needed, and they relieve you of the effort of interviewing candidates and the complications of paying Social Security. In addition, such employment agencies are usually licensed by the state and their employees often must be bonded (ask the agency about this).

Health care or nursing agencies can provide aides who do light housekeeping and errands such as shopping. People they send are likely to be accustomed to your situation; that is, they will expect to find things around the house without being shown. These aides can give you personal care, such as emptying bed pans or washing hair. Cost per hour can vary, so shop around.

Firms listed under "House Cleaning" are generally a bit less expensive. They can dispatch people to do heavier housework, but seldom personal care. Shop for price and for a firm that concentrates on regular help, not one-time jobs.

Other sources of help are:

- **Referrals from friends**

- **Classified ads**

- **The Employment Development Department in your state**

- **Student placement offices in high schools and colleges**

- **Newsletters and bulletin boards of church, community, and charitable agencies, like those dealing with the disabled, senior citizens, or women**

- **Neighborhood organizations in some low-income areas**

- **Some ethnic organizations**

The last four can be low-cost, but a response may come too late or never.

If you spend any time in the hospital, ask to see the hospital's specialists before you go home on bedrest—social workers, perinatologists, neonatologists, physical therapists. Ask if the hospital has a support group for people in your situation, whether books are available, and what other resources exist.

If You Have Other Children

Bedrest at least gives you time to spend with your children. Although you will be unable to do many things that you ordinarily would do for and with them, your cuddling and attention will help make up for what they are missing. Establishing some routines, such as a regular story time, will help children feel that their lives are less disrupted.

Keep special toys and projects by your bed, such as favorite toys, a model being built, or board games. Read to your children or have them read to you. Older children can help with anything from massaging your feet to cooking or running errands.

Children may become angry, withdrawn, or display their fears and sense of "losing" you. Normal apprehension about the coming "rival" can become magnified. Explaining the situation and being reassuring may help, but may not completely solve the problem. If you need someone to talk to about children's behavioral problems, you can call one of the parental-stress hotlines described in the section "Counseling, Information, and Referral."

You will need childcare for children so young that they must be picked up or dressed. It may be easier to stay in bed if older children, too, are cared for by someone else. Non-profit, state-supported referral centers can shorten your "shopping" for childcare of all kinds: day care, latchkey programs, babysitters, or overnight childcare.

Financial aid for childcare is extremely limited, but if you are in need, ask the referral lines:

1. Are respite care funds available? (This is temporary care in emergencies.)

2. Is any other financial aid or subsidy available? (There usually are long waiting lists.)

Some parental-stress hotlines have funds for short-term respite care (up to 48 hours). If you are on welfare, you may be able to get financial help with childcare; ask your social worker about federal "Title 20" funds.

As a last resort, you can contact the county's Social Services Department, Children's Protective Services, for foster placement of children. Although the agency's goal is to reunite families, this does involve police and a court proceeding. If you can, get advice from someone familiar with the system before taking this step.

Things to Have

This list goes from near necessities to luxuries that may be worthwhile only if you were considering buying them anyway.

✔ An "eggcrate" mattress cover to make your bed or couch feel softer. If you get one in the hospital, you can bring it home with you. Or try a hospital supply store for this and other useful supplies, such as elbow guards to protect your elbows, which you will use to move around while lying down instead of using abdominal muscles.

✔ Lots of pillows. For lying on your side you need at least three: for head, back, and between your legs. A large angled pillow is a good backrest for sitting up (ask your doctor how far you can sit up).

✔ The largest bedside table you can find. Use a card table or a coffee table from another room.

✔ Bedside storage, such as low shelves or stacked crates, for books, food, medicines, and craft projects.

✔ Water pitcher, carafe, thermos, ice bucket, ice chest or cooler. Having some of these will save you trips for food or drink.

✔ Plastic basins, lots of washclothes and towels, for washing in bed. (You may be able to take some supplies from the hospital, if you are hospitalized before bedrest at home.)

✔ A tray table or hospital-style table for meals.

✔ For taking medicines, an alarm clock or a watch with a second hand for taking pulse, and enough alarm clocks to set one for each time you need to take medicine at night (some clocks allow for two different settings); a small book light; pill boxes or extra prescription bottles so that your medicines are accessible where you spend time (but out of reach of children).

✔ A firm footboard and headboard for your bed, to push against if you are able to do isometric exercises to maintain your circulation and muscle tone. You may be able to jerry-rig these by wedging a board between mattress and frame.

✔ Stickers and safety bars in your tub or shower and possibly by the toilet, if you are unsteady on your feet.

✔ Mild indigestion remedies and/or mild laxatives, *as recommended by your doctor or midwife.* You may be able to avoid indigestion by eating small quantities, or avoid constipation with natural remedies such as prunes, high-fiber foods, and drinking lots of water.

✔ Plants, flowers, music, or new decorations in your bedroom can help your mood, as can attractive robes and housedresses. A bird feeder you can watch is a delight.

✔ Subscriptions to magazines.

✔ A cordless telephone or long cord so that the telephone can reach you. A list of phone numbers, including doctor, pharmacy, friends, work colleagues.

✔ A bell to ring when you need something, or a home intercom if your room is far from others (some people use one later to listen to the baby). An intercom to the front door can also be useful.

✔ A tape player and cassettes are easier to manage from the bedside than a record player.

✔ A bedroom TV set, subscription to cable or pay TV, or a rented or purchased video player (VCR) to show films at home.

✔ A home computer and software for games and programming.

Things To Do

Being restricted to bed can be quite difficult. By keeping busy in bed it is easier to stay quiet, you feel better about yourself, and you worry less. We have listed a range of activities. Try some of these or others, but don't set arbitrary goals; medicine may sap most of your energy, and you may accomplish less than you expect.

First of all, continue your uterine monitoring each day. It is a physicial necessity and something to do!

Keep a calendar to mark the progress of the pregnancy. Have a small celebration at the end of each week. You may find this a morale booster, and you'll see concretely how much you are accomplishing. (Some women prefer to ignore calendars at first, and just let the days pass—especially if put on bedrest quite early, with several months to go.)

Puzzles—jigsaw, crossword, or those found in books—can pass hours you spend alone or with children, spouse, and friends.

Sketching with colored pens or pencils can be done with

inexpensive notebooks and aren't as messy as watercolors, oils, pastels, or charcoal.

Crafts—knitting, crocheting, and embroidery are easier to manage than sewing. Inexpensive booklets can teach you to knit or crochet. Books of patterns for almost anything—including layettes and baby toys—cost only a few dollars. Other possibilities are leather craft, basketry, and weaving small things. If these aren't your style, try building a model of some sort, possibly with an older child or your partner. Avoid crafts that have large or heavy parts, use many different kinds of materials, require physical effort, or involve water or other spillable liquids.

Organize—for example, make a family photo album, build a recipe card file from newspapers, magazines, or cookbooks from the library. Mend things.

If you are allowed, a bath can be quite relaxing. However, be sure *first* to get specific instructions from your doctor on whether baths or showers are allowed. (If so, how often, how warm, how much standing, etc.)

Keep a journal or record your thoughts on tape. This can help you deal with feelings. Write anything you always wanted to write—poetry, fiction, or letters to friends, politicians, editors.

Learn the "natural history" of the area outside your window. Do squirrels or other animals visit, and when? What do they eat? Where do they sleep? When do different birds sing?

Get public library materials. Most libraries will deliver and pick up books, tapes, or records. Check such departments as Outreach Services, Bookmobile, Mobile Library, or Handicapped Services in the listing for your local public library in government listings in the white pages.

Have someone read to you.

Learn by TV. Educational programs on public television can teach you anything from fancy cooking to flying. If you are put to bed near the beginning of a semester, call your local public television station for a schedule and information on how to get college credit TV courses.

Take a correspondence course. Contact a nearby university for a correspondence course catalog. The Independent

Study Catalog, listing credit correspondence courses from around the nation, is available from the University of California Berkeley Extension, Independent Study, 2223 Fulton Street, Berkeley, CA 94720, for $6, plus $2 additional for first-class mailing. A typical UC course costs around $150, not including textbooks.

Learn a language or a computer language. Books, records, and tapes are available from public libraries or stores.

Volunteer. Two possibilities for volunteering are telephone fund raising and participating in "friendship lines," regular telephone calls to other shut-ins. During political campaigns, your help in telephoning prospective voters would be welcome. To find volunteer opportunities, contact your favorite arts, civic, or charitable organization, or call the United Way Volunteer Bureau or a volunteer center.

When arranging visits from friends and family, follow your instincts as to when and for how long. Have people call first, and be honest about good and bad visiting times.

Arrange some romantic time with your partner—for example, a catered candlelight dinner in bed (the caterer can be your neighborhood deli), or a date to watch a special movie on the television or VCR.

Bedrest Exercise (*Only* as recommended by your doctor)

The goal of a "bedbound" exercise program is to limit the undesirable effects of limited physical activity—on muscles, bones, and blood circulation—without causing increased uterine activity or strain. Be sure to check with your health care provider *before* beginning any exercise program.

Your doctor can prescribe visits from a physical therapist (hospitals that have programs in high-risk pregnancy often have physical therapists experienced with bedbound pregnant women). Some medical insurance plans will at least partially cover such visits or cover a one-time consultation with a physical therapist to set up an exercise program for you.

Even with medical approval, watch the effect of each exercise. Some women on bedrest can do isometric exercises; others find that even those rather mild exercises cause contractions. Breathe regularly while exercising. Avoid any

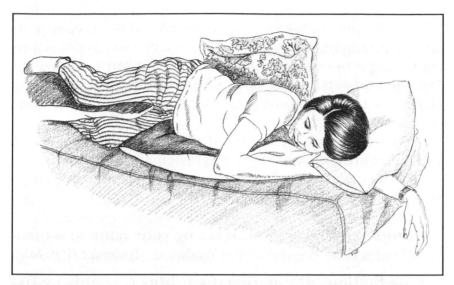

Figure 16 — Use lots of pillows for good support while lying down.

exercise that uses muscles in the abdominal region, that puts you in a squat-like position, or that involves holding your breath while exerting effort.

Do not lie flat on your back. Remember to put a small pillow or folded towel under one hip so you will be tilted to your side (preferably the left side—*see figure 16*). This prevents the full weight of the pregnant uterus from compressing the major veins and arteries supplying your uterus and legs.

Try to exercise at times when you have the least uterine activity. Before beginning your exercises, make sure your bladder and blowels are empty and you are comfortable and relaxed. The exercises are to help you through your bedbound period, not create more problems, so listen to your body. *Don't do too much!* And, if any exercise increases contractions, stop doing the exercise immediately.

Getting Through the Night

Insomnia (inability to sleep), a problem in many pregnancies, can be aggravated by bedrest. Tension, indigestion or other discomfort, side effects of medicine, and the fact that you just aren't getting tired in the daytime, all can make it more difficult to sleep.

A book light that clips to a book and lights only the page

will let you read or take medicine without waking your partner. Furthermore, you may need to wake up several times during the night to take medication. If you can learn to wake up to a soft wristwatch alarm, so much the better. But set a backup alarm clock for each time you must take your medicine, just in case.

Warm milk, a warm shower (if allowed), or gentle massage at bedtime are tried-and-true ways to help you relax and sleep.

Two mental techniques that can help you relax and fill time as well as sleep are:

- **Progressive relaxation: relaxing your body one muscle at a time** (*see Relaxation Technique, Appendix B, p. 143*).

- **Meditation: eliminating disturbing thoughts by fixing your mind on some pleasant or neutral thing, commonly a word or set of syllables.**

There need be nothing mystical or religious about these techniques. All can be learned on one's own, through books or tapes. You can easily modify instructions to suit bedrest— for example, by lying on your side instead of on your back, or skipping the deliberate contraction of muscles before you relax them.* Or you may be able to develop your own method of relaxing.

Bedside Bargain Hunting**

You may need to shop for maternity and/or nursing clothes, baby things, ordinary household needs, and gifts. Catalogs and sale ads make this easier and more economical than you might think.

Subscribe to your local newspaper. Watch sale ads and clip coupons. Many people find that the coupon savings more than pay for a newspaper subscription.

Specialized magazines and newspapers for mothers of young children are full of ads and mail-order offers. The

---

*Two tapes, #20033 Meditation and #20040 Deep Relaxation, are available from *Psychology Today* magazine: Psychology Today Tapes Dept. A1040 P.O. Box 770, Pratt Station Brooklyn, NY 11205.

**Specific items, stores, catalogs are listed on these pages and in Appendix C for your convenience. This list is not exhaustive, and we are not recommending or endorsing those included here.

national monthly magazines *Mothers Today, American Baby,* and *Baby Talk* are distributed free in doctors' offices and stores that sell infants' things.

Collect catalogs and compare their prices with those advertised in newspapers. Although many items can be bought by mail, sight unseen, others probably should be checked by a friend or partner. For example, a "bargain" crib may not be sturdy enough because it lacks steel reinforcement. Some useful catalogs are listed in Appendix C.

Childbirth Preparation "Classes"

Don't give up on childbirth preparation. Hospitals with high-risk pregnancy programs may be able to recommend someone who knows how to adapt the training to your condition and who will teach you in your home. Books are also available.

Non-Strenuous Outings

If you are on "limited" bedrest, and your doctor approves, you might try:

- **Movies, concerts, or theater as long as seats are comfortable and you need not stand in line or climb to a balcony.**

- **Restaurants with comfortable chairs, in off-hours when service is faster.**

- **Major museums, which supply wheelchairs free of charge.** (Call in advance to find out how to get one.)

- **If you can borrow or rent a wheelchair, your partner can push you on a stroll. Try the zoo or an accessible park near your home. Contact the administering agency for more information on parks in your area.**

Financial Aid

Employee benefits. If you were employed when you were put on bedrest, ask about the firm's disability and maternity leave benefits. You probably will use a combination of both.

State disability. If you were employed when you went on bedrest, you probably qualify for state disability benefits. Call your state's Employment Development Department or Disability Insurance Division (listed in the government section of the white pages). Someone can pick up and return the necessary forms, which must be filled out by you and your doctor. Do this as soon as possible, as waiting times are at least three weeks.

WIC food program. If your income is low (whether or not you were employed) you can apply for vouchers for nourishing food for yourself while you are pregnant and for your baby after delivery. Contact your local WIC program, listed in the government section of the white pages under county health departments. You need someone who knows you well and whom you can trust because, in addition to having someone pick up the forms (which must be signed by you and your doctor), you will need someone who can discuss your report on your diet with a representative of the program, and someone to buy your groceries regularly, whose name can be on your WIC vouchers along with yours.

AFDC, Food Stamps, Medicaid (called MediCal in California). If you have little or no means of support, you may qualify for Aid to Families with Dependent Children (welfare benefits), Food Stamps (coupons for food only), or Medicaid. If you want or think you are eligible for only one or two of these programs, ask about applying separately. If possible, get advice from someone familiar with the welfare system (perhaps a hospital social worker or a public health nurse) before applying.

Apply through your county Social Services Department or its district office nearest you (these are listed in the government section at the beginning of the white pages of the telephone book). A representative can pick up an application for you. At the same time, call your county Social Services Department to find out whether your representative can take it to the office to be evaluated.

Processing or even obtaining an appointment can take up to 45 days, so ask about retroactivity. Once you are on AFDC, you may be eligible for a variety of benefits, including childcare or psychological counseling.

Counseling, Information, and Referral

Months of enforced bedrest can take a toll on any expectant mother, and on her partner, who has to work outside the home and do the pregnant woman's share of the household chores, perhaps go without sleep, and care for and support her.

Check in your area for groups providing telephone support and information for expectant and new parents (ask at the hospital; check yellow pages under "Health Services"). Talking to people in your situation can help. Ask your doctor, midwife, or hospital for names of other families who are or have been in your situation. Some hospitals have formal support programs of this kind.

For support in coping with children, you can call parental stress hotlines or telephone numbers. Primarily set up to lessen child abuse, these groups also will advise you on other child-related problems. Some can help with emergency short-term childcare.

General information and referral is available from United Way Information and Referral. Information and referral on disability and local services for the disabled are available from local Easter Seal Society offices. Find these numbers in your telephone book.

In the hospital, the social worker can give advice on practical and psychological matters.

County health department nurses will visit your home to advise you on medications and on arranging your life during bedrest and after the baby is born. Call your county health department or district office. Fees generally are adjusted to income, or one visit is free.

Members of the clergy will make home visits for counseling. For names of professional counselors who will come to your home, contact organizations for the disabled.

How to Eat Well When You Must Rest in Bed*

Many women who must restrict their activity during pregnancy find that eating well can be a problem for the following reasons.

*Adapted from materials by Barbara Abrams, University of California at San Francisco.

- **It is difficult to buy, prepare, and eat food while in bed.**
- **Medication used to treat preterm labor may decrease the appetite.**
- **Some women find that inactivity can cause constipation, which is both uncomfortable and may make eating less appealing.**
- **Some women find that the combination of constant bedrest, along with anxiety about "Will my baby be all right?" decreases appetite and weight gain.**
- **Other women find the combination of less activity and the boredom of being in bed all day increases food cravings and intake so that too much weight gain occurs.**

These are very real problems. It is important to remember that your baby is depending on you for nourishment. The quality of your baby's growth, both physically and mentally, can be affected by what you eat now.

You need foods to supply two kinds of nourishment:

Extra Energy (Calories): Fuel for your own body, for the baby's growth, and energy to utilize nutrients.

Extra Nutrients: Building blocks that actually become the baby's body. These include protein, vitamins, and minerals.

A vitamin supplement supplies some of the nutrients you need, but not the most important ones: calories and protein. Thus, while vitamin pills provide some nutritional insurance, they do not serve the same function as food.

You should eat: A variety of dairy products, protein foods, whole-grain breads and cereals, fruits and vegetables. If you have not received a prenatal diet guide, ask your health care provider for one.

It is important that you eat well now, especially if your baby may come before term. These weeks are a critical growing period for your baby.

If you are on medications, find out whether you need to follow a special diet (such as one with less sugar or more potassium) to counteract side effects.

Coping with Food Problems While on Bedrest

Food Purchase and Preparation

List the foods that you need bought. Be specific. Plan menus consisting of foods that:

- are non-greasy, not messy

- need little or no refrigeration

- need little or no preparation

- could be included in a "bag lunch"

Some simple nutritious foods are:

- hard-boiled eggs

- fruit

- yogurt

- cheese slices

- nuts

- vegetable sticks

- cottage cheese

- cream soups

- sandwiches on whole-grain bread

- milk shake

- bran muffins

- crackers and peanut butter

- small cans of juice

Try non-greasy take-out foods like pizza, Chinese and Japanese foods, burritos, barbecued chicken. When possible, eat take-out foods that are not fried.

Food Storage at Bedside

- Keep a pitcher of water for fluids. Remember, you need at least four to six cups of liquids per day.

- Use a thermos for soups, milkshakes, fruit-yogurt drinks.

- Have an ice chest for cottage cheese, milk, sandwiches, cheese slices, vegetable sticks, yogurt.

Poor Appetite—Low Weight Gain
- Try to relax.

- Eat at regular times.

- Eat small, frequent meals.

- Choose foods that give the most nutrition for the calories, such as milk, hard-boiled eggs, milkshake, yogurt.

- Drink fluids between rather than during meals.

- Write down what you eat. Try to identify when and what you could add throughout the day, such as peanuts, trail mix, milkshake.

- Schedule visitors at mealtime for company.

- Call your nutritionist for advice on your diet.

Excessive Appetite—High Weight Gain
- Eat at regular times.

- Eat more low-calorie, high-nutrient foods, such as raw vegetables, fruit, low or non-fat milk, low-fat yogurt.

- Write down what you eat. Try to identify when and what you could delete throughout the day, such as cookies or other high-calorie snacks.

- Call your nutritionist for advice on your diet.

Constipation
- Eat high-fiber grains such as bran and wheat germ.

- Drink a lot of fluid, such as water and fruit juices.

- Drink hot water with one teaspoon of lemon juice three times a day.

- Eat more raw fruits and vegetables.

- Eat at regular times.

- Ask for a stool softener if dietary measures are not producing results.

Nausea
- Eat five or six small meals a day. Never go for a long period without food.

- Drink fluids between rather than with meals.

- Eat lightly seasoned foods. Avoid foods cooked with pepper, chili, and garlic.

- Avoid greasy and fried foods.

- When you feel nauseated between meals, drink small amounts of apple juice, grape juice, or carbonated beverages.

- Get some fresh air, if possible; for example, set up a chaise lounge outside.

CHAPTER

6

Cerclage

Two types of medical treatment are currently most common for threatened preterm delivery. One treatment is a surgical procedure—called a cerclage—in which a stitch is placed around the cervix in an attempt to keep it closed. The other type of treatment uses medications to stop excessive uterine activity (*see Chapter Seven*). The decision to use one or the other of these treatments—or a combination—should depend on an analysis of the woman's particular symptoms and reproductive history.

Labor is usually a dual process of uterine contractions and cervical changes, leading to the opening (*dilation*) of the cervix—which allows the baby to pass through (*see Chapter One*). In some pregnant women, the cervix dilates too early, without excessive uterine contractions. That is, the cervix seems to open "on its own," as if this part of the uterus were not strong enough to hold the growing fetus. This condition is sometimes called *cervical incompetence* or *cervical insufficiency*. We do not know why some women have a "weak" cervix; however, the following characteristics have been suggested as contributing factors.

- **Abnormal cervical structure—congenital** (born with this structure) **or from previous surgery** (such as a cone biopsy, in which part of the cervix is removed).

- **Abnormally short or misshapen cervix or, perhaps, abnormal cervical tissue** (such as in a woman exposed to the hormone diethylstilbestrol (DES) before birth—that is, while still in *her* mother's womb).

- **Scars in the cervix due to healing of tears that occurred during previous deliveries.**

- **Injury to the cervix from multiple forceful dilation during previous therapeutic abortions.**

It is often difficult to know whether a woman's cervix should be considered weak or insufficient to hold through a pregnancy. For instance, a short or misshapen cervix—whatever its origin—is not necessarily a *weak* cervix. In a nonpregnant state, a woman may appear to be likely to have an incompetent cervix during pregnancy if an x-ray (*hysterosalpingogram*) shows problems or if a thick dilator can easily be passed through the cervical opening. However, these indications have *not* proved to be valid in predicting an incompetent cervix during pregnancy.

The diagnosis of cervical incompetence is usually made on the basis of the woman's past pregnancies and/or signs that develop during the current pregnancy. Did she lose one or more pregnancies between 13 and 26 weeks of pregnancy, without unusual uterine activity or following a "silent" rupture of the membranes (the bag of waters breaks in the absence of labor)? Does her obstetrician now detect cervical changes during a pelvic exam, without evidence of excessive uterine activity when monitored?

If you have reason to suspect you may risk cervical incompetence, discuss with your physician whether pelvic exams should be done during the second and third trimesters of your pregnancy to check for cervical changes. Practitioners disagree about the risks and benefits of such exams, since the exam itself could contribute to uterine activity or introduce infection.

How Is Cerclage Done?

If a woman is diagnosed as having a weak cervix, her doctor may recommend a cerclage.

A cerclage is a strong stitch placed around the cervix in a circle, to support the cervix and keep it closed (*see figure 17*). In nearly all cases, the cerclage is inserted through the vagina. There are two different types: the McDonald and the Shirodkar cerclage (named after the physicians who developed the specific technique). The difference between the two involves how far up on the cervix the stitch is placed and, therefore, how extensive the actual surgery must be.

Some obstetricians use the Shirodkar method on women who have had a McDonald's cerclage that did not hold, or who have a cervix that appears too short for a successful McDonald's suture. If you are considering a cerclage, discuss the pros and cons of each method with your obstetrician. You may also want to ask how much experience she or he has had with each; if possible, find an obstetrician who has done these procedures many times.

Placement of the stitch can be done under general or

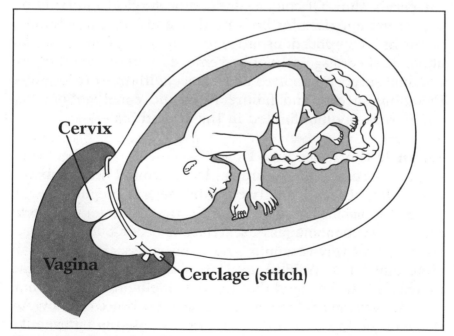

Figure 17 — Cervical cerclage.

regional anesthesia, depending on the preferences of you and your obstetrician. Usually, women stay in the hospital for a couple of days following the surgery to be certain there is no unusual bleeding, uterine activity, or sign of infection. Occasionally, the obstetrician wants you to take antibiotics or tocolytic medications (*see Chapter Seven*) during and after the surgery to prevent infection or uterine contractions. Anything you take, of course, also goes to the fetus. You may want to discuss these issues with your obstetrician.

In uncomplicated cases, the cerclage is removed close to term but before labor begins in order to prevent damage to the dilating cervix.

On very rare occasions an *abdominal cerclage* is considered. This cerclage is placed higher on the cervix and can be inserted only through an incision in the abdominal wall. Two major surgeries are needed—first, to put the cerclage in, and second, to perform the cesarean delivery that is then required. An abdominal cerclage is considered only if the cervix does not extend far enough into the vagina or if previous cerclages inserted through the vagina have "come out" or failed to hold the cervix shut. Of course, this major surgical intervention carries greater risks for both mother and baby; in addition, if further complications arise during the pregnancy, the abdominal cerclage cannot be removed without another abdominal surgery. Reported experience with this procedure—including success and failure rates and complications encountered—is quite limited in the United States.

When Is the Procedure Done?

In most cases, the suture is placed around the cervix between the thirteenth and twentieth weeks of pregnancy. The reason for placing the suture after the first trimester is to allow for an early spontaneous miscarriage to occur. Such a miscarriage is relatively common, and is often associated with an abnormal fetus. Waiting until after the first twelve weeks increases the likelihood that the developing fetus is normal.

If the diagnosis of incompetent cervix is based on previous pregnancy history, the cerclage is often inserted as a preventive measure, even before signs of cervical change appear.

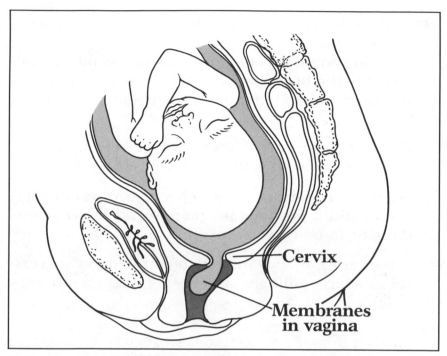

Figure 18 — Bulging of bag of water into birth canal: "Hourglass membranes."

Weighing the Risks and Benefits

As with any medical intervention, the cerclage does carry risks for the pregnant woman and the fetus. These risks include: 1) the usual complications of anesthesia; 2) significant bleeding from the cervix; 3) infection around the suture; 4) uterine irritation caused by the procedure, which can lead to excessive uterine activity and may ultimately result in preterm labor and delivery.

If a cerclage is inserted properly and before significant dilation of the cervix has already occurred more than 2 centimeters, the likelihood of these complications is quite low—up to 85 to 90 percent of these pregnancies will progress long enough for the baby to survive. However, if the cerclage is placed after the cervix has already dilated more than 2 centimeters, or if the amniotic membranes are bulging through the cervix into the vagina (*hourglass membranes, see figure 18*), the success rate is much lower.

You and your health care providers, of course, want to avoid unnecessary or inappropriate use of cerclage. If a cerclage is recommended to you, you may want to ask such questions as:

- **Do your symptoms or *indications* suggest that a weak cervix is the likely problem?** (For example, if you are also experiencing uterine contractions, the cerclage could be torn out.)

- **Have less "aggressive" interventions been tried** (such as bedrest, reduced physical activity, etc.)?

- **Does a pelvic exam show signs of cervical change, and/or did a previous pregnancy end in what was thought to be cervical incompetence?**

- **Is the cervix already dilated too far to make successful cerclage unlikely, and/or are the membranes bulging?**

Deciding to put in a cerclage is frequently a "judgment call," reached after assessing the various factors in a patient's history and present condition. Be sure to discuss with your obstetrician the risks and benefits *in your particular case.*

CHAPTER

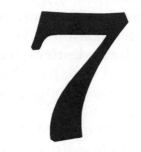

Tocolytic
Medications

The second major type of treatment for preterm labor uses medications in an attempt to stop uterine contractions. These medications are called *tocolytic* substances, or "labor-inhibitors." Before describing specific medications most commonly used in the United States, a few general comments may be helpful.

Most tocolytic medications reach the uterus through the circulating blood. The blood also carries these substances to other parts of the body, including the heart, kidneys, brain, and stomach. Although the desired target for preterm labor medications is the uterus, the medications also have an effect on other parts of the pregnant woman's body, called *maternal effects*. In addition, when these medications reach the uterus, they cross the placenta to the baby, causing *fetal effects*.

These consequences are known as *side effects*—that is, effects of the medications beyond the desired result, which is to relax the uterus. Side effects vary in how long they last, how serious they are, how unpleasant they feel, and how well they can be managed by the patient and the obstetric staff.

Individual women vary in how they respond, physically and emotionally, to these medications.

Women frequently ask, "How will these medications affect my baby?" Research to answer this question has been done with animals and, to a limited extent, with humans. Some of the medications discussed here have been used for over 25 years and quite a bit is known about both maternal and fetal effects. Less is known about other medications. Additional research is needed to learn more about both immediate and longer-lasting effects of these drugs.

Despite research, some uncertainty always remains about presently unknown risks that could be identified in the future. One fact in this regard is especially important: Tocolytic medications are *not* given during the first three to four months of pregnancy when the fetus is most susceptible to potential harm from drugs and other exposures; rather, tocolytics are usually given *after* 20 weeks of pregnancy, which is beyond the most sensitive period of organ development. In existing studies focusing on short-term effects, no major abnormalities have been reported in newborns after treatment with tocolytic medications.

As with any medical intervention, the decision to use tocolytic medications requires weighing the benefits (gaining time for the growing baby) against the risks (undesirable side effects and possible unknowns) for mother and baby. This evaluation needs to be tailored to each pregnancy: What is the woman's health? Are there reasons a particular treatment should *not* be given (*contra-indications*)? How well could the baby do if there is no treatment and a preterm delivery does occur (usually related to how many weeks of pregnancy have already passed)? We discuss these questions further in the coming pages.

If you do receive medications to stop preterm labor, close supervision by an experienced obstetric staff is essential. These medications are very strong. Although most women can take them without experiencing serious complications, you and your health care provider do need to watch for any side effects that may require a medical response; for some women, the dosage must be lowered and, in a few

cases, the medications stopped.

This chapter contains basic information about the medications used most often to stop preterm labor. We hope this background will help you discuss your own circumstances with your physician.* Our experience suggests that if women are told what side effects to expect, and how to handle them, they are usually able to tolerate the treatment very well if, in fact, this treatment becomes necessary.

We can describe here only a few of the more common side effects. There are others, experienced by fewer women, which you can learn more about from your practitioners. Most of the side effects mentioned appear during the beginning of treatment by injections. After about 12 to 24 hours of treatment, these effects generally become milder. When taking the medication in pill form, the side effects are even fewer, although it is still important to watch for any unusual reactions.

You may find it useful to talk over the various issues and choices with your physician *before* any problem arises that could result in use of these medications. That way you can reach preliminary decisions, and feel comfortable with a tentative "plan."

Beta-Adrenergic Medications— Adrenalin-like Substances

In this country, the medications most commonly used to stop preterm labor are called *beta-adrenergics*. This name comes from "adrenalin," because these medications are similar in chemical structure and effect to the hormone adrenalin, which our bodies produce naturally. The beta-adrenergics (also called *beta-mimetics*) have been known to obstetricians for more than 25 years. The various medications within this group have similar characteristics and similar success rates in stopping preterm labor. This group of medications includes: ritodrine (brand name: Yutopar), terbutaline (brand name: Brethine, or Bricanyl—often used to treat asthma), isoxsuprine (brand

---

*Our focus is on the two types of tocolytics presently used in Northern California and at the hospitals affiliated with our San Francisco preterm birth prevention program. If your physician uses other substances, be sure to ask about expected side effects and advantages/disadvantages of that medication for you and your baby.

name: Vasodilan—also used to treat vascular disease), solbu-
tamol, fenoterol.

How Beta-Adrenergics Are Administered

At the present time, no single treatment program has been
identified as the most successful. If a woman is in very active
preterm labor, most obstetricians begin these medications with
injections—either into the vein (*intravenous*), into the muscle
(*intramuscular*), or into the fat under the skin (*subcutaneous*).
Injections are used to reach high and effective concentrations
of medicine quickly, so that the preterm labor can be stopped
as soon as the diagnosis is made. Since side effects can sometimes be significant, treatment by injections *must* be started
in the hospital, and *only* where an experienced staff is available
to manage potential complications.*

After labor has been controlled for 12 to 24 hours, treatment with pills can be started. The pills are then taken at
regular intervals and continued at home. In some cases, excessive uterine activity returns, and the woman must go back
to the hospital for treatment by injection.

To estimate whether the amount of medication appears to
be adequate, practitioners often use the maternal pulse rate,
since increased pulse rate is a common effect of these substances. If the pulse rate is slow (below 90 beats per minute
for most pregnant women), and uterine activity is excessive,
this may be considered a sign of too little medication. On the
other hand, if the pulse is more than 110 to 120 beats per
minute for long periods of time, the dose should probably be
reduced, especially if there are no contractions.

If you are taking a beta-adrenergic medication, it is helpful
to learn how to take your own pulse, record it, and report it
to your practitioner. In this way, maintaining a proper dosage
will be easier. The best times to measure your own pulse rate
are 20 to 40 minutes *after* taking the medication, and a second time *just before* taking the next pill. Ask your practitioner

---

*Some physicians do begin treatment with pills if they think a woman may be in very early or
mild preterm labor. These cases involve a judgment about whether the symptoms actually represent
preterm labor, and how aggressively they should be treated. The goal, of course, is to minimize cases
where medications are prescribed unnecessarily, whether by pill or injection, while catching early true
cases of preterm labor.

to teach you how to take your own pulse and record the pulse rate.

If you do require beta-adrenergic medication, the treatment should continue uninterrupted. These medications generally stay in the blood circulation for only a short time, and after two to four hours their level in the blood is so low that they lose effectiveness. If you take the pills only when you feel contractions, you might miss uterine activity (especially when asleep or preoccupied by other activities), thereby increasing the risk of preterm delivery. It is very important to take the pills at regular intervals, day and night, usually every two to four hours.

Be sure to discuss thoroughly with your practitioners just how your treatment will proceed and how it will be supervised. Below are the instructions given to women in the San Francisco program. These instructions reflect a fairly standard routine for taking oral medications (pills):

> After uterine activity has been controlled in the hospital for 12 to 24 hours by injections of medication, treatment can usually be changed to pills. Initially you will take the pills every two to four hours, and probably remain on bedrest during the first 24 hours. (Your individual medication plan will be worked out with your physician.) If everything remains quiet, the following day you may increase your activity slowly—for example, get up for the bathroom and shower.

> If uterine contractions do not recur during the next 24 to 48 hours, you may go home. At home, it is important that you continue taking the pills, day and night, at regular intervals. Your activities at home will need to be limited. Your physician will tell you how often to take your pills, and show you how to check your pulse rate. She or he will describe the amount and types of activity you can do at home. Before leaving the hospital, you may want to make arrangements so you can rest well at home. You may need help with work around the house. If you have other children, you may need help with childcare. (A hospital social worker may be able to help with these arrangements.)

> You will continue to take the pills at home, every two to four hours, until you reach 37 weeks of pregnancy. Even though you are taking medication, it is possible for labor to start again.

Therefore, you should continue to monitor for contractions and notify your physician if there is an increase in uterine activity.

Be sure to take your pulse before each dose of medication. Your pulse rate should be between 90 and 110 beats per minute. If it is faster than this (more beats per minute), do *not* take another pill. Notify your practitioner, and ask when (or whether) another pill should be taken. She or he may change your dosage according to your pulse rate. In general, we want your pulse to be either: between 90 to 110 beats per minute or 15 to 20 beats above your usual pulse during pregnancy, that is, your "baseline" rate before treatment. If your pulse is consistently below 90 beats per minute, your physician may prescribe more medication (unless your usual, baseline rate was very low). If your pulse is consistently too high, the dose may be reduced.

Since these medications must be taken regularly, day and night, set your alarm before you go to sleep—to wake up and take your pill It is not necessary to check your pulse throughout the night if the rate has been stable and within the designated limits.

If contractions do become regular and do not decrease with the pills, bedrest, and fluids, you may need to return to the hospital. Injections may be restarted if the pills are not controlling uterine contractions. It can feel very discouraging to have to receive injections again; but try to feel encouraged that you recognized your contractions and are taking steps needed to keep them under control.

Known Side Effects of Beta-Adrenergics

Effects on the pregnant woman (see figure 19). As mentioned above, one common side effect of beta-adrenergic medications is an increased pulse rate. These substances cause the heart to beat faster while at the same time causing the uterus to relax. These medications affect other parts of the body as well. Figure 19 lists the major maternal side effects, describing both mild and severe forms. When possible, the average estimated frequency with which these side effects occur is given—that is, out of 100 women being treated approximately how many will probably experience the particular side effect. The side effects occur most prominently with intravenous administration, and generally subside after the first few days.

Maternal Side Effects of Beta-Adrenergics

The side effects listed (and approximate percentage of women who experience them) occur mostly with intravenous administration of the medication.

Organ System	Mild	Severe
	(Notify physician if sympton persists)	*(Notify physician at once or go to hospital if receiving medication at home)*
Heart	Rapid pulse (more than 90%)	Rapid pulse if woman has heart disease before the pregnancy
		Congestive heart failure (less than 5%)
		Strong chest pain (less than 5%)
	Palpitation, irregular beats (15–20%)	Palpitation if woman has heart disease before the pregnancy
Lungs	Slight shortness of breath (15–20%)	Severe shortness of breath
Stomach & Intestine	Nausea, vomiting (20–25%)	
	Constipation (20–25%)	
		Intestinal paralysis (less than 5%)
Blood	Elevated sugar levels (temporary)	Elevated sugar levels with diabetic condition
	Decreased potassium levels (temporary)	
Skin	Skin feels warm (10–20%)	
Neurologic (central nervous system)	Tremor, slight shaking (20–35%)	
	Sleeplessness, restlessness (less than 5%)	
	Headaches (15–25%)	Prolonged, persistent migraine headaches
Kidneys	Water retention, less urine, thirst	

Figure 19 — Maternal side effects of beta-adrenergics.

Effects of Beta-Adrenergics on the Baby	
On fetus	Increase in heart rate
On newborn	Abrupt decrease in blood sugar levels after birth (temporary)
	Decrease in blood calcium levels after birth (temporary)
	Slight decrease in blood pressure (temporary)
	Relaxation of intestines (temporary)

Figure 20 — Effects of beta-adrenergics on the baby.

An experienced obstetric staff will help reduce the chances of harmful side effects by doing certain tests before and during treatment. Tests include EKGs to measure cardiac (heart) effects, and blood and urine tests to measure various metabolic effects. Do not hesitate to ask your practitioner for further information about the different tests and what the results indicate. If side effects become too prominent, your practitioner can reduce the dosage or switch to another medication.

A very important point: Women who already have heart disease, diabetes, or hyperthyroidism should *not* take beta-adrenergic medications. For these women, the side effects of this type of drug are too dangerous (that is, the risks outweigh possible benefits). Be sure to tell your practitioners if you have any of these health conditions or any other that might make beta-adrenergic medication undesirable. A different type of treatment will be chosen. (For further discussion of "contra-indications"—reasons *not* to take medications—*see below*).

Effects on the baby (*see figure 20*). These substances reach the baby's circulation a few hours after the woman starts the medication. The effects appear to be similar to those seen in the mother, although less pronounced. "Fetal effects" can include:

1. a slight increase in the baby's heart rate;

2. an increase in blood sugar levels, if there is an increase in the mother's levels;

3. a decrease in potassium level, if a decrease occurs in the mother.

These medications disappear from the bloodstream very quickly after stopping the treatment. If beta-adrenergic therapy is stopped 12 to 24 hours before delivery, the drug level in the baby's bloodstream is very low by the time the baby is delivered. Harmful effects have not been reported in these babies.

Any newborn whose mother was treated with beta-adrenergics should be watched for side effects which, though rare, may require medical attention: changes in the blood sugar of the newborn (most frequently, very low blood sugar levels); low calcium levels; relaxation of the intestines; lowering of the blood pressure. In most cases, these problems have no known long-term consequences if handled appropriately in the newborn; babies who have been followed over several years show completely normal development.

Magnesium Sulfate

Magnesium sulfate has been known to obstetricians and other practitioners for several decades. However, "mag-sulfate" has been used primarily to treat certain high blood pressure disorders in pregnancy (also called *toxemia* of pregnancy, *preeclampsia, pregnancy-induced hypertension*). We now know that magnesium sulfate can stop preterm labor. In fact, a major advantage of magnesium sulfate is that it appears to have a relatively low number of side effects (*see figures 21 and 22*). In addition, it is possible to monitor accurately the levels of this medication in the bloodstream, making it easier to keep a safe and effective dosage. The fact that this medication is very familiar to practitioners provides additional safety since they are likely to have experience handling its side effects.

For women who cannot be given beta-adrenergic injections or who cannot tolerate the side effects, magnesium sulfate is usually a good alternative. Some obstetricians think this medication should be used in most cases of active preterm labor, with beta-adrenergics used as the alternative, if needed. (Magnesium sulfate is also a less expensive substance than the beta-adrenergics.)

Maternal Side Effects of Magnesium Sulfate

Organ System	Mild	Severe
	(Notify physician if sympton persists)	*(Notify physician at once!)*
Stomach & Intestine	Nausea, vomiting (less than 5% of women)	Intestinal paralysis (less than 5%)
Blood	Decrease in blood calcium level (less than 5%)	
Skin	Warmth (temporary)	
Neurologic (central nervous system)	Sleepiness	Suppressed breathing (rare, only if toxic dose given)

Figure 21 — Maternal side effects of magnesium sulfate.

Effects of Magnesium Sulfate on the Baby

On fetus	Occasional variability from normal heart rate pattern
On newborn	Decrease in blood calcium level (temporary)
	Decreased muscle tone (temporary)

Figure 22 — Effects of magnesium sulfate on the baby.

The major disadvantage of magnesium sulfate is that it cannot be given effectively in pill form. Its use, therefore, is limited to treatment by injection. Once the uterine contractions have been stopped, and oral medication can be used, it is necessary to switch to the beta-adrenergic pills described previously. In addition, it is not yet clear whether magnesium sulfate is as effective in stopping contractions as the beta-adrenergics.

Known Side Effects of Magnesium Sulfate

Effects on the pregnant woman. Figure 21 lists maternal side effects observed when using magnesium sulfate.

Effects on the baby. In cases where delivery occurred soon after treatment (12 to 14 hours), lowered calcium levels in the blood, decreased muscle tone (limpness), and decreased alertness have sometimes been reported (*see figure 22*). These effects in the newborn are quite rare, and do not last long if diagnosed and treated promptly. In such cases, no long-term harmful effects have been reported.

Other Substances

Over the years, various substances have been used in attempting to stop preterm labor. Medical knowledge and practice change, and new methods replace those that were once standard treatments. Today, physicians and scientists are exploring still newer medications and other alternatives that may be safer and more effective than the treatments presently used.

Physicians are free to use any medication available, and at times they do try new things, especially in cases where the usual treatment is not working or is contra-indicated. Furthermore, medical professionals differ in their interpretations of research findings and in their opinions regarding the safety and/or usefulness of particular substances. In some places, the latest information has just not become a part of the treatment program. We list below some substances that you may encounter, including some that have been used in the past and others that are future possibilities being used experimentally in some places.

Do not feel hesitant to ask your physician for more details about these treatments for preterm labor, if they are prescribed. For example, what is the latest information about immediate and long-term side effects for you and your baby? What are the success rates with this particular substance? Why is she or he choosing this type of medication over other alternatives?

Alcohol (Ethanol): In the past, alcohol was often given intravenously to women in preterm labor; in some cases, it seemed to stop uterine contractions. Side effects of alcohol treatment, however, can be significant for both mother and baby. For the pregnant woman, these effects are similar to intoxication from drinking alcoholic beverages. For the baby, long-term *fetal effects* can include those now identified in cases of chronic alcohol consumption (known as *fetal alcohol syndrome*), including impaired physical and mental development. Because of the side effects, most practitioners no longer consider alcohol to be an appropriate treatment for stopping preterm labor.

Prostaglandin-Inhibitors—Indomethacin, Naprosyn (antiinflammatory agents): The production of a hormone called *prostaglandin* is involved in the process of labor and delivery. Prostaglandin-inhibitors, which decrease production of this hormone, have been used successfully in the United States and in other countries for the treatment of preterm labor; they are given primarily as pills and occasionally as rectal suppositories. Although these medications can stop preterm labor contractions, their safety for the baby has not been demonstrated. Prostaglandin-inhibitors are not very popular with practitioners in the United States because so little is known about effects on the baby.

Progesterones: During pregnancy the placenta produces large amounts of the hormone progesterone. Progesterone-like medications can be given in a natural or synthetic form. Recent research indicates that large doses of natural progesterone (administered by injection or rectally) can stop preterm labor. However, since the number of patients in those studies was relatively small, more experience is needed before we can feel more certain about effectiveness and long-term safety. We do know that hormones given *early* in pregnancy, such as estrogens (for example, diethylstilbestrol) and synthetic forms of progesterone (progestins) could cause health problems for the offspring. Therefore, concern remains generally about giving hormones to pregnant women.

"Calcium Entry Blockers": A new type of medication to stop contractions has been used on a very limited basis by some physicians. These substances block the action of calcium on the uterine muscle, an action known to be involved in contractions. Although these medications have been used more widely to treat heart disease, they have not been used previously during pregnancy. Only in recent years have physicians in Europe applied this medication to preterm labor with varying success rates. In the United States, experience is very limited, and more research is currently underway. Effects on

the fetus are not known and need much further study. Although not approved specifically for use in stopping preterm labor, this medication is available to physicians. Some believe these drugs will be the treatment of choice for stopping preterm labor in the future. If your physician wishes to try such substances, be sure to discuss the known and unknown risks, as well as evidence of effectiveness.

Another Medication Your Physician
May Wish to Use—Corticosteroids

Corticosteroids (cortisone-like steroid hormones, such as betamethasone or dexamethasone) are not given to relax the uterus and stop preterm labor, as are the tocolytic medications described above. However, we mention them here because they are often administered to women in preterm labor in conjunction with tocolytic therapy.

Corticosteroids given to a woman in preterm labor are thought to speed up the maturation of her baby's lungs before birth, by enhancing production of a substance called *surfactant* (a baby produces surfactant on its own in sufficient amounts during the last weeks of a full-term pregnancy). For premature infants a major complication and cause of death is respiratory failure (*respiratory distress syndrome*) which results from immaturity of the lungs at the time of birth. Corticosteroids are administered to the mother if a preterm delivery is anticipated. In the San Francisco program, approximately one-half of the cases diagnosed as preterm labor are quickly controlled and corticosteroids are not needed. In the other half, where a delivery may occur, corticosteroids are sometimes used. They are most effective if given at least 24 to 48 hours prior to birth.

Since these potent hormones do affect other organs, there is some disagreement over their risks and benefits for the baby. Use of lung maturation medications should be limited to cases where likely benefits outweigh known and unknown risks. As a pregnancy progresses, the risk of respiratory distress syndrome following delivery decreases; the likelihood of benefits from corticosteroids, therefore, also decreases. Some practitioners think the benefits of using corticosteroids are greatest between 28 and 33 weeks of pregnancy. A test of amniotic fluid by amniocentesis can help determine whether the un-born baby's lungs are mature (as with any medical procedure, the test itself does carry a small risk—in this case, of increasing uterine activity even more).

Contra-Indications: When Tocolytic Medications Should *Not* Be Used

When considering any medical intervention, one of the first questions is: "Are there reasons this patient should *not* have this treatment?" Just as there are symptoms or indications your practitioner looks for to identify the need for a medication or surgical procedure, there are also *contra-indications*—reasons against treatment.

As an informed patient who may experience preterm labor, you should have a general idea of the contra-indications for tocolytic medications so you can discuss your own care with your physician, should the need arise. Reasons not to use tocolytic medications fall into two categories:

1. *Situations in which preterm labor absolutely should not be stopped.* That is, no type of treatment for stopping preterm labor should be attempted, and the baby should be delivered. These are cases in which prolonging the pregnancy poses a greater risk to the mother and/or baby than does the baby's premature delivery. Some examples are:

- **The mother has severe high blood pressure, or hypertension, of pregnancy** (*eclampsia*).

- **There is a severe premature separation of the placenta from the uterine wall, disrupting the supply of nutrients and oxygen the placenta normally carries to the baby inside the uterus.**

- **There is severe maternal bleeding.**

- **There are signs of infection inside the uterus.**

- **The baby is much smaller than normal throughout the pregnancy** (*severe intrauterine growth retardation*).

• **The baby has died inside the uterus or there is a fetal abnormality diagnosed before birth that eliminates any chances for survival after birth.**

2. *Situations in which treatment* may *not be recommended.* Many cases of preterm labor fall into this category, in which a final decision requires very careful evaluation of the advantages and disadvantages of treatment for mother and baby, and a judgment about the degree of risk associated with prolonging the pregnancy.

Weighing the Risks and Benefits of Tocolytic Medications

As the previous section suggests, most cases of preterm labor call for a judgment about the advantages and disadvantages of using medications, for both the pregnant woman and her baby. In other words, you and your family, as well as your practitioners, need to ask: "Do the likely benefits of using the medication outweigh the risks that also come with this treatment?" In some cases, the decision is fairly easy; in others, the judgment is more difficult because the risks and benefits appear more "even." Here are a few basic considerations to help you begin thinking about your own circumstances.

1. Gestational age of the baby: How far along is your pregnancy? How premature will your baby be if born now? How long can delivery probably be delayed and what are the likely gains for your baby during that time?

In general, the benefits of tocolytic medications are clearest when preterm labor begins many weeks before your due date. If a baby is born between 24 and 32 weeks of pregnancy (term is beyond 37 weeks), she or he certainly may survive, but could have significant and perhaps lifelong complications related to prematurity. During those earlier weeks, then, the benefits of keeping the baby inside the womb—of gaining time for the baby to mature—are considerable. The risks to an infant born at 26 weeks are much greater than risks to an infant born at 35 weeks of pregnancy, not only in terms of whether the baby will survive, but also regarding the likelihood of prolonged hospitalization and possible handicaps. Most of the known risks of tocolytic medications are to the mother. These risks are the side effects—physical and emotional—of these substances. The newborn infant experiences very few observable side effects from the medication. Follow-up studies of children born after prenatal exposure to tocolytic medications are currently in progress. Preliminary information does not show any long-term harmful effects as the children grow older.

2. Medical condition of the mother: Because of known maternal effects, careful evaluation of the pregnant woman's medical condition is essential before starting tocolytic medications, whether by injection or pill; ongoing evaluation of side effects must continue throughout tocolytic treatment. Be sure to tell your physician if you have any health problems, such as heart disease or diabetes. (If a problem is being followed by another practitioner, your obstetrician may wish to speak with him or her.) Your obstetrician needs this information when you first see him or her, in order to provide you with appropriate prenatal care. If you later experience preterm labor, *remind* your physician, so that the proper treatment can be selected.

3. Emotional impact of tocolytic medications: Experiencing preterm labor and the need for treatment can certainly cause anxiety for a pregnant woman and her family. For the woman, this anxiety is increased by tocolytic medications, because their side effects include feelings of anxiety and restlessness. You and your physician need to remember that these medications may cause you to feel uncomfortable—physically and emotionally—particularly during the first one to four days of treatment. In most women, this discomfort will then decrease. However, once treatment of preterm labor is started, you may need to continue some type of medication, bedrest, and/or restricted activity until you have reached approximately 37 weeks of pregnancy. This time period may be quite long. In addition to a commitment on your part, you will need help and support from family, friends, and your health care providers.

When weighing the risks and benefits of tocolytic medications, your ability to cope with this situation must be one consideration. Remember, as your pregnancy progresses, the "balance" of risks and benefits changes. Decisions about tocolytic medications at 25 to 28 weeks of pregnancy involve different factors than decisions at 34 or 35 weeks. Even if you are receiving tocolytic medications, you can talk over with your physician the question of how long treatment should continue—again, giving careful thought to your condition and the possible outcomes for your baby.

Signs to Look for During Treatment

If you do receive tocolytic medications, you can play an important role in observing your own condition, so that your treatment is geared to your particular needs. During tocolytic therapy, you should watch for two possibilities that may require a change in the dosage and/or type of medication. Your role is particularly important when you are at home, on pills, although you can keep a watchful eye even in the hospital, and let a doctor or nurse know if you detect any problems.

Possibility #1: *Signs that preterm labor may be returning.* Remember to monitor regularly for uterine activity just as if you were not receiving treatment. Taking these medications does not ensure that preterm labor will never return. Our experience suggests it is better to err on the side of caution. Therefore, continue to monitor to be sure contractions do not become excessive.

Possibility #2: *Signs of side effects needing attention from your practitioner.* We have already described the need for you to take your pulse while on tocolytic medications, as a way of estimating whether the dosage is correct. If *at any time* you feel aware of your heartbeat, you should check your pulse. If your pulse rate is faster than 120 beats per minute for several hours, or if you feel that your heart skips beats or beats irregularly, even if the rate is slower than 120 beats per minute, notify your practitioner . If you just feel that your pulse is fast when it is between 90 and 120 beats per minute, record your pulse rate and try to ignore what is sometimes called "heart- awareness" (*palpitation*) associated with beta-adrenergic medications. If you are not certain about your pulse or heartbeat, call your practitioner.

If *at any time* you have chest pain or significant shortness of breath, notify your practitioner at once! If you have been pregnant before, you may be familiar with the usual shortness of breath that women feel during the last three months of pregnancy. If you are not sure whether you are feeling *unusually* short of breath, check with your practitioner.

Occasionally, headaches occur during oral tocolytic therapy. If a headache persists, contact your practitioner for advice about taking common remedies such as tylenol or nonmedicinal techniques.

Remember, if you cannot reach your practitioner but think your condition should be checked, you can always go to your hospital or clinic.

Some side effects of tocolytic medication require patience and/or mild, common "remedies." For example, since tocolytics relax the intestinal smooth muscle, as well as the smooth muscle of your uterus, you might suffer from occasional nausea and even vomiting. If tocolytic medication is taken in combination with bedrest, constipation may become a major problem. No pregnant woman at high risk for preterm labor should use enemas at home under any circumstances, because an enema may increase uterine activity; however, since constipation may also increase uterine activity, we recommend using mild stool softeners such as Metamucil or Colase. If the problem is with hard stools that hurt during bowel movements, you may be able to use glycerine suppositories. Before trying any of these over-the-counter (non-prescription) remedies, please be sure to discuss them with your practitioner!

Other side effects reported during tocolytic therapy—such as feeling warm, jittery, tired, or nervous, having insomnia, mood swings, or short tempers—generally need no special treatment. Support and reassurance by family, friends, and your practitioner may be helpful.

If You Do Feel Restless and Anxious

Restlessness and "anxiety attacks" are side effects some women experience when given these drugs. Since there is no specific antidote for this side effect, we can only offer you the knowledge that:

- **these feelings are largely a result of the medication;**

- **you are taking this medication for an extremely important reason; and**

- **these side effects usually lessen with time, and will disappear as soon as the medication is stopped.**

In our experience, one of the most helpful ways of coping with tocolytic medication is to talk with other women who are undergoing this treatment at the same time or have recently done so. Ask your practitioner if you could be introduced to one or two such women. It often helps to know that you are not alone in this special world of "preterm birth prevention." And another comforting thought: Preliminary reports from programs aimed at preventing preterm birth show good success rates. If the medications are started early in preterm labor and taken consistently at appropriate doses and intervals, reports indicate that 70 to 80 percent of women diagnosed in preterm labor will have term or near-term deliveries.

Extended Hospitalization

As we described previously, after preterm labor is diagnosed, and tocolytic medications are determined to be necessary, the usual procedure is to begin with injections in the hospital, then change to pills; the pills are continued at home. In a few cases, however (approximately 10 to 15 percent), oral medication does not successfully control uterine contractions. For reasons we do not understand thoroughly, excessive uterine activity returns for some women taking only pills. In this situation, long-term treatment by injection may be necessary. This treatment must generally be done in the hospital, with the woman on bedrest (an I.V. line or *catheter* will be placed in the arm, allowing continuous intravenous medication). If you do require this type of tocolytic therapy, treatment will begin in the hospital's labor and delivery unit. When uterine contractions have been controlled, you may be moved to a different unit for a longer stay. Depending on how far along

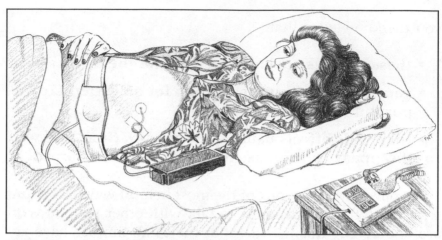

Figure 23 — Home management of preterm labor.

your pregnancy is, several weeks of hospitalization may be necessary. As always, the medication must be administered, and side effects monitored, by an experienced obstetrician and nursing staff. The health of two patients—mother and baby—must be carefully guarded, and treatment tailored to the individual case. You need to tell the doctors and nurses any symptoms you are feeling while in the hospital (such as nausea, blurred vision, tightness or pain in your chest, pain at the I.V. site, a feeling of heaviness).

No one can claim this experience is a pleasant one, but remember, it does not last forever!

New Techniques in Management of Preterm Labor

Recent research in preventing premature birth has introduced new ways to detect preterm labor in its earliest stages and to treat preterm labor once it has been diagnosed. The use of a home electronic monitor has been valuable in recording uterine contractions for women at increased risk of delivering prematurely. It is a small belt that holds the monitor around the waist and then connects to a small portable recorder. It detects contractions that often are not felt by the woman herself. The data are stored and then can be transmitted over the telephone for immediate evaluation. The monitor may be valuable in making an early diagnosis of premature labor (*see figure 23*).

A new way of delivering the medication terbutaline is by slow infusion under the skin via a small, portable pump. This delivers a very small dose on a continuous basis and can be used at home as well as in the hospital. The terbutaline pump may make the management of preterm labor easier and can help more women continue their pregnancy at home.

In the Hospital
We describe below some of the people, equipment, and procedures that are likely to be a part of a longer-term hospital experience for treatment of preterm labor. Although there will be variations at different hospitals, the following pages can give you a general idea of what to expect.

Upon Your Arrival

- You will be welcomed and admitted by a labor room nurse. At first, you will be carefully monitored to determine the frequency of your contractions and the rate of your baby's heartbeat.

- You will be requested to lie down on your left side, a position that often helps to slow down contractions.

- Your own private doctor, a hospital staff physician, or a nurse will conduct a physical and pelvic examination, at which time a cervical culture will be taken to test for possible infection.

- You will be given a blood test and a urine test.

- An electrocardiogram will be performed to monitor your heart's activity.

- An I.V. will be administered to give you additional fluids and to infuse medication to slow your contractions.

- You may be given an injection of betamethasone immediately and again in 18 hours to help your baby's lungs mature.

- You will continue to be monitored very closely. Your vital signs, including blood pressure and heart rate, will be checked frequently.

Monitoring

You will be on the monitor continuously. To help you understand your preterm labor, your nurse will explain how to read the monitor.

There are two parts to the monitor (*see Chapter Four*):

- The ultrasound transducer, which records your baby's heart rate (also called *Fetal Heart Tones*, or *FHT*).

- The "toco" or *tocodynamometer*, which detects and records your contractions.

If your baby is small and very active the monitor cannot always pick up the heart rate. Therefore, a nurse may periodically listen to the baby's heart. Sometimes your own heartbeat is also picked up by the monitor, but it can easily be distinguished from the baby's heartbeat, which is usually much faster. The gel used on the transducer is very cold and, sometimes after long use can cause some redness or itching. In most cases, the baby's heart rate does not need continuous monitoring, and this part of the machine can be turned off.

Your uterine contractions, on the other hand, should be monitored continuously. Because it is extremely important to know when you're having contractions, you can help keep the toco in place. When you change position, the toco must often be readjusted.

If you experience contractions that are not picked up by the monitor, please notify your nurse. She or he will help differentiate between the baby's movement, gas pains, and contractions. Together, you can determine the best location for the toco.

Bedrest

Bedrest is one of the most essential components of your treatment. When you are settled into your bed, you may be requested to lie on your side with your head slightly lower than your feet to elevate your hips (known as the *Trendelenburg position*). In addition, you will be encouraged to remain on your left side as much as possible. If the bed becomes uncomfortable, ask about obtaining an "egg-crate" mattress.

Bedpans

Because you are confined to bed, you will be required to use bedpans for emptying your bladder and moving your bowels. Your nurse will be happy to assist you and provide you with as much privacy as possible. All your urine will be measured and tested. Try to keep your bladder empty. A full bladder can stimulate contractions. Your doctor will probably order a stool softener to prevent constipation. We also encourage you to include roughage (fresh fruits and vegetables) in your diet.

Daily Food Selection

During your hospital stay, you will receive a regular menu to choose from. Select foods that are high in protein and calcium, and rich in fiber, such as bran, salads, and fresh fruit. Avoid coffee, tea, cola drinks, and other forms of caffeine. You may have food brought in from home.

Fluid Intake

With certain I.V. medications (such as ritodrine) your fluid intake must be limited in order to avoid side effects. Therefore, you may not be able to drink as much as you would normally like. The total amount of fluids allowed during a 24-hour period ranges from 1800 cc to 2000 cc (about eight glasses), including the amount you receive in your I.V. For example, if you are receiving 30 cc an hour in your I.V., that means you can only drink approximately 1200 cc, which is equal to about five glasses of fluids per day. Your nurse will be happy to help you devise a daily plan for fluid intake.

Bed Baths

Although your nurse is available to assist with your daily bed bath, you may discover that you can manage most of it by yourself. Not only that, your daily bath offers a good opportunity to get some exercise.

Bed Weight

You will be weighed each morning on a bed scale to watch for excessive fluid retention.

Blood Tests

After the first 24 hours, your blood may be drawn once each morning for testing.

Ultrasound

Your physician may order a sonogram, which will be performed either in your room or in another room to which you will be wheeled on a flat gurney. A simple and painless procedure, the sonogram uses high-frequency sound waves to determine the size of the baby's head (*biparietal diameter*, or *BPD*), the amount of amniotic fluid, the position of the baby and placenta, and as a guide during amniocentesis.

Amniocentesis

Amniocentesis is a procedure in which a sample of amniotic fluid is removed and tested for bacteria and to judge the baby's lung maturity. The presence of two chemicals, lecithin/spingomyelin (L/S) and phosphotidyglycerol (PG), helps to determine whether the baby's lungs are mature enough to function outside the womb. These particular tests do not reveal the sex of your baby. If amniocentesis is ordered by your doctor, you will be requested to sign a written consent before the procedure is performed. Please discuss amniocentesis with your doctor if you have any questions about the test or its risks and benefits.

Planning Your Day

If you are hospitalized for a long period, try to schedule your time. Although the morning is often busy with hospital routines, it's helpful to plan the rest of your day. Set aside specific times for making phone calls, receiving visitors, doing exercises, taking a nap, reading, watching TV, or working on a craft. A well-structured day will not seem as long (*see Chapter Five*).

The Multidisciplinary Health Care Team

In addition to the obstetric nursing and medical staff of the labor and delivery or the after-delivery unit, several other specially trained professional staff are available to help you.

- A physician from the Newborn Intensive Care Unit staff will visit you to discuss any concerns you may have about your baby. In addition, family members are welcome to tour the Newborn Intensive Care Unit.

- If your hospital is associated with a medical school, you may see residents, interns, and/or medical students who are assisting in your care.

- A dietician is available to assist with menu selection or to suggest alternative food choices.

- A physical therapist can create a daily exercise program for you.

- A social worker is available to discuss and help find solutions to problems associated with your hospitalization. Additionally, she or he will help you plan for returning home.

A few hints from women who have remained hospitalized on medications for several weeks:

- Be aware of your medication schedule. Patients can help assure that the correct dose of medicine is given at the correct time.

- You may find that some nurses are better than others at inserting I.V. needles (that is, it hurts less!). Try to have one of the more experienced nurses do it whenever possible.

- Some hospital routines may be bent a bit, especially if you are a long-term guest, such as food, visiting, number or time of routine tests. It doesn't hurt to ask about possible changes that will make you more comfortable.

- Have visitors bring food you like. It may provide a boost to your tastebuds *and* your morale.

- If your fluid intake is restricted, try sucking ice cubes and eating more fruits. They last longer and are refreshing.

- You need to let people at the hospital know if something prevents you from sleeping at night or from resting comfortably during the day. In such cases, don't be concerned that you are complaining or "causing trouble"—see if something can be worked out. Also be sure to let the nurses and doctors know if you feel contractions that are not showing up on the monitor!

Being in the hospital can make you feel that things are completely out of your hands, but that need not be true. Remember, you are the same person you were before entering the hospital. You know about your own condition, and can still make decisions about your care. Patients can refuse treatments or procedures, but do need to know the pros and cons before doing so. Talk with the doctors and nurses, and remain as involved as you wish to be.

8

If Your
Baby Does
Come Early

Unfortunately, efforts to prevent preterm delivery are not 100 percent effective. It is important to remember, however, that *delaying* a delivery for several weeks can be extremely important, even if the actual delivery is still preterm. For some women, preterm delivery cannot be avoided. In many such cases, we cannot identify a specific reason. It is *not* something the pregnant woman did or did not do, nor is it a result of her attitude. There is, for instance, a small proportion of women who just do not respond to the available medications—the contractions persist. We want to discuss briefly a few issues about delivery, as they relate specifically to a preterm birth, so that you know what decisions may be necessary. You may want to give these issues some thought, just in case.

At Which "Level" Hospital Should Delivery Occur?

Even before the actual preterm delivery, there is a question of where the delivery should take place. A hospital's

Obstetric and Newborn Services are assigned different "levels" of care (Level I, Level II, and Level III) according to the types of treatments available and, therefore, the complexity of problems that can be handled. At Level I hospitals, services are limited primarily to low-risk obstetrics patients and full-term infants who may need only minor help just after birth (for example, temporary aid with breathing). If a sick newborn needs more intensive therapy, she or he must be transferred to a hospital with a Level II or III nursery, where greater resources are available. Level II nurseries can handle a limited number of moderately sick newborns; however, if very tiny or sick babies require complex treatment, they need to receive care in a Level III newborn nursery (sometimes called a *tertiary* center).

If it appears that a mother with a problem pregnancy will deliver prematurely, and her hospital is not Level III, many practitioners think it is best to transfer the mother to a Level III center before the delivery. The alternative is to wait, and transfer the newborn premature infant to a Level III hospital if the baby does need more complex care. The potential advantage of *maternal transport* (that is, transferring the still-pregnant woman before delivery) to a Level III hospital is that neonatal specialists, with expertise and equipment for very sick newborns, are available immediately, when the baby is delivered. If intensive, complex care is needed, there is no delay in obtaining sophisticated diagnoses or treatments not available at a lower-level hospital. In addition, risks of the transport itself for a newborn premature infant are avoided. Another advantage of maternal transport is that mother and baby are at the same hospital after the birth; if the newborn is transferred following delivery, the mother remains in the hospital where she delivered.

A disadvantage of maternal transport is that the Level III hospital may be far from home. Delivery may occur in unfamiliar surroundings, with a feeling of isolation from family, friends, and the expected supportive environment. Quite often, the practitioner who provided prenatal care will not be able to deliver the baby at the Level III center. In other words, maternal transport requires a bit of adjusting for the mother, and for her family and friends.

As always, the decision about where to deliver depends upon your particular case, and evaluations made by you and your practitioner. Knowing that you are at risk for preterm labor, you may want to discuss the following questions with your obstetrician: 1) What level of care can be provided at the hospital where you plan to deliver? 2) If this hospital is Level I or II, should you go to a different hospital—with a Level III nursery—if preterm labor does develop? 3) If you deliver at a Level I or II hospital, where would your baby be taken if she or he does need to be transferred after birth? 4) If you are to be delivered at a different hospital, who are the practitioners who will take care of you and deliver your baby?

What Type of Delivery?

Although the methods available during a preterm delivery are essentially the same as those at full-term, there are some special considerations due to the baby's prematurity. As a general rule, a premature baby should be delivered in the least traumatic way possible. "Least traumatic" means a gentle delivery, with the smallest amount of manipulation and the smallest amount of medication, so that there is very little interference with the baby's functioning after the birth.

Vaginal birth or cesarean section. Most practitioners think that a premature baby can be delivered vaginally if the baby is

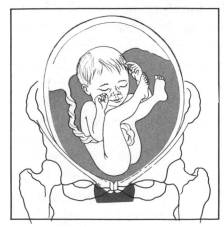
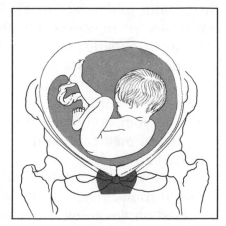

Figure 24 — Baby in breech position.   *Figure 25—Baby in transverse position.*

coming with head first, there is no evidence of *fetal distress* (indicated through monitoring of the baby's heart rate), and there are no reasons for a *cesarean section* (surgery to remove the baby through an incision in the abdomen and uterus) based upon the mother's condition. Some practitioners do not agree with this approach; they think a C-section is always safer and more gentle for the premature baby. You may wish to discuss this issue ahead of time with your physician, so that you understand her or his viewpoint and reasons.

If the premature baby is not head-down—for example, lying sideways or *transverse*, or with legs or buttocks coming first (*breech*)—a C-section is usually done (*see figures 24 and 25*).

Pain Medications

Premature babies are generally more sensitive to medications that relieve the mother's discomfort during labor and delivery than are full-term babies. The premature infant takes longer to metabolize and get rid of these medications, mainly because the liver and kidneys are not as ready to handle such substances as are those of a mature baby. During labor and delivery, therefore, the goal is to provide relief to the mother by giving: 1) substances that will be cleared from both maternal and fetal circulation by the time delivery takes place (such as morphine or demerol); or 2) regional anesthesia that numbs one part of your body, and affects the baby only minimally (regional anesthesia includes spinal anesthesia, epidural anesthesia, and pudendal block). Regional anesthesia is administered by an injection into the spaces outside your spinal column, or outside and around the nerves that conduct pain sensations to the brain from various regions of the body (such as the uterus, the cervix, the vagina). With regional anesthesia, you are alert during labor and delivery, while a particular region in your body feels no sensation of pain. Very little of this type of medication enters your blood circulation or that of your baby.

As with the decision about mode of delivery, the choice of medications given during labor and delivery must always be based on weighing the risks and benefits for you and for your baby.

Forceps

Forceps are a pair of instruments (*see figure 26*) that fit on both sides of the baby's head just behind the eyes and cheek bone. Some practitioners believe that a "forceps delivery" may help protect the soft skull of the premature infant from the pressure of the pelvic muscles during the final stages of labor. In most cases anesthesia (local, regional, or general) is used.

Vacuum Extraction

This technique uses a relatively small (one and one-half to two-inch diameter) instrument built in the shape of a cup. The cup is applied to the head of the baby and adheres to it by vacuum. It can help in delivery efforts by gently pulling during your contractions. If used, the baby's head may temporarily look rather misshapen. Again, practitioners differ in their views of whether and when this use of a vacuum is appropriate.

Episiotomy

During this procedure, an incision is made at the outer part of the vagina (between the lower part of the vaginal opening

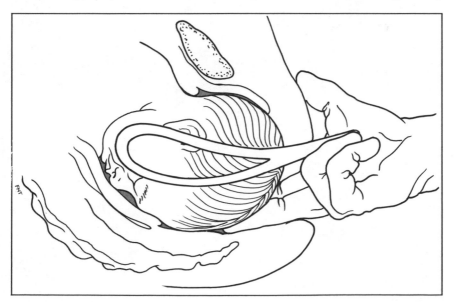

Figure 26 — Forceps delivery.

and the rectum) in order to enlarge the vaginal opening and prevent tears in the area by enhancing a smooth delivery. Some practitioners feel that an episiotomy (which can be done under local anesthesia) may be valuable for delivery of the premature infant because it reduces pressure of the pelvic muscles against the baby's soft head.

You may want to discuss the above procedures with your physician; opinions do differ about the value, or risk, of these manipulations during preterm (or full-term) delivery. There are no "answers" from medical studies.

CHAPTER

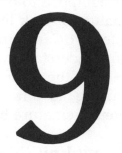

The
Premature
Infant

A baby born preterm is usu-
ally taken immediately from the delivery room to the special
nursery. This experience may feel upsetting to the new parents;
however, their baby is receiving the attention and care she
or he needs at the moment—a thorough examination to determine how premature her or his development appears to
be* (remember, "preterm" refers to dates, "premature" to how
able the baby is to function outside the womb), as well as a
quick response to health problems that may be identified. Most
infants born prematurely, even those who are ill, will recover;
the majority live normal lives. But being born prematurely
does increase the risk for medical and developmental problems
in the early childhood years.

Not all babies who are born preterm need intensive care.
Some preterm infants weighing more than four pounds require

---

*In order to acknowledge that the baby may be either male or female, but to avoid continually
using the awkward phrases "he or she" and "him or her" when referring to the baby, we alternate using
male or female pronouns throughout each section of this chapter.

117

little or no special treatment. In this section, we describe the type of nursery that is equipped to provide the highest level of care for very premature or sick infants—Level III, often called the Newborn Intensive Care Unit (NBICU). The following pages will help you understand what is going on there; who all the people are, what the equipment is, and what your role can be. After describing the nursery, we provide a general idea of health conditions premature babies may experience.

Newborn Intensive Care Unit (NBICU)—What Is It?

The intensive-care nursery is an area where newborn babies can receive special care. Usually between two-thirds and three-quarters of the infants in the NBICU are there because of prematurity. The others are babies who were born at full term, but have a health problem needing special care. Some of the babies in the NBICU are very tiny and very sick; others look big and healthy, and need to spend very little time there. The NBICU is unique because it is equipped specifically to deal with the problems of sick newborns, with special equipment sized for tiny babies. A highly trained staff of doctors, nurses, technicians, and other personnel skilled in dealing with newborns and their families is available around the clock.

The NBICU is a warm, noisy, brightly lit and very busy place. Several pieces of equipment and many staff members are involved in caring for each baby, and there are several babies in each room. So, it is often crowded and there is very little privacy. (For example, at Children's Hospital of San Francisco, the NBICU has 20 nursery beds and more than 100 staff members working.) Phones ring, alarms go off, people talk—there is a constant feeling of tension. All of this can seem overwhelming when added to your concern about your baby.

For the parents it helps tremendously to be able to identify all of the different people and their different jobs. Here is a key to "who's who" in newborn intensive care:

Nurses are the backbone of the intensive-care nursery. Many nurses with varying years of training may work with your baby. *Registered nurses* (R.N.s) have completed two to five years of medical training and have passed a state examination. In addition, most R.N.s have special training and experience in neonatal (newborn) care. They perform most of your baby's care—for example, starting intravenous lines, drawing blood for tests, giving medications, as well as changing diapers and feeding your baby when you are not there.

Licensed vocational nurses (L.V.N.s) or licensed practical nurses (L.P.N.s) have 18 months or more of training; they work under the supervision of an R.N.

Some hospitals use *clinical nurse specialists* and *neonatal nurse practitioners* to help with neonatal care. These nurses have received extra training, usually through a master's degree program beyond their training as a registered nurse. Their role varies in different hospitals; they may serve as educational resources to parents and staff, or they may function much like interns and residents (*see below*) in providing care directly to babies.

Physicians specializing in the care of children also staff the NBICU. Most Level III NBICUs are in teaching medical school hospitals where physicians train to be specialists. The doctors receiving medical training work under the supervision of a *neonatologist* (newborn specialist). A neonatologist is a *pediatrician* who specializes in the care of newborn infants. Usually, several neonatologists share the workload. Each month one will take a turn as the "attending physician"—the doctor who is the main supervisor in charge of care for all the infants each day. At night, the "attending physician" shares with his or her partners the responsibility for being available ("on call"). Physicians working under the supervision of the neonatologists are:

1. *Fellows*—fully trained pediatricians who are completing extra years of training to be neonatologists. They perform many of the medical procedures in the NBICU. They also teach and do research within the medical school. Fellows provide additional help at night to the interns and residents.

2. *Interns* and *residents* (also called "house officers") are qualified physicians who are training to be general pediatricians. An intern is in the first year after medical school; residents have already been interns. They spend one to two months each year for three years in the NBICU, and then move

on to other parts of the hospital. One of the interns or residents stays in the hospital throughout the night to take care of immediate problems. They work on a rotation schedule—one or two times per week each house officer works for 36 hours straight. Be aware that this individual may appear grumpy and rumpled the next day.

The doctor caring for your baby in the hospital will usually not be providing your regular well-baby care when you go home. This ongoing care will be the job of your own family's pediatrician. In the hospital, your pediatrician will usually participate in decisions with the neonatologists, but most of the actual care is done by the hospital's neonatal staff. If you and your doctor live far from the hospital, your doctor should be in frequent communication with the hospital physicians, who will keep him or her informed about your baby's care. If you have not chosen a pediatrician for your baby yet, do so now—yes, before the baby is born (*see Chapter Two*).

While your baby is still in the hospital, there will be *technicians* who are also directly involved in daily care. These individuals are trained to perform specialized tests, such as taking x-rays, drawing blood, performing ultrasound or EEG examinations, when such tests are requested by the doctors. Most NBICUs also have respiratory therapists—people specially trained to assure that equipment needed to help your baby breathe, or to give extra oxygen, is ready and in good working order.

Other personnel with specific skills may be called in from time to time for any additional needs your baby may have: *developmentalists* (specialists in infant development); *pediatric neurologists* (pediatricians whose specialty is the baby's central nervous system and brain); *pediatric cardiologists* (heart specialists).

And, finally, there is a staff person who is not directly involved in caring for your baby but is there *for you*. A *social worker* is available to help answer questions about insurance, provide information about support services (for example, help at home, transportation, parent support groups, financial support for special needs), or just to talk if the going gets rough.

With so many different people taking care of your baby,

you may not know to whom you should speak when you have questions. You may find it less confusing to talk with the same few staff members each day—for example, the resident, or fellow, or your baby's primary nurse. As you get to know the individuals, it will probably become easier to ask your questions and get the answers you need. Remember, however, that you can always ask to speak with a supervising physician or nurse about your baby. In some instances, you may have to be a bit insistent—but that is your right!

Getting to Know Your Baby:
The Parents' Involvement in Care

Being a parent in an intensive-care nursery is difficult both physically and emotionally. Many parents are puzzled by their intense reactions to all of it. They may have strong, even physical, reactions to walking into the NBICU, such as dizziness, nausea, sometimes panic.

There are ways to help yourself be more comfortable. First, wear cool clothes. The room is kept quite warm for the babies (around 75 degrees), and you will be required to wear a hospital gown over your street clothes when you are in the unit.

Second, ask what the visiting rules are and when the best times to visit are. Most NBICUs allow parents to visit as frequently and for as long as they wish; however, there may be limits on other visitors because of limited space and concerns about infection. A special request concerning visiting can often be arranged ahead of time.

Try to learn the daily routine; some times of day are always more busy and confusing than others, so you may want to plan your visits to avoid those times. The doctors meet together regularly each day to exchange information and discuss treatment plans for all the babies in the unit. These discussion meetings are called *rounds*. The nurses have similar meetings to exchange information (every eight hours in most hospitals) as each shift changes and new nurses come on duty. During rounds and changes-of-shift are *not* the best times for parents to ask questions or to find quiet time to spend with their baby. See if you can work around these meetings.

More difficult than physical arrangements, of course, are

the emotional feelings you may have. You will probably ride an emotional rollercoaster as you wait for your baby to get better. There will be highs and lows, good days and bad. If your baby is very premature, it may sometimes feel as if bad weeks are followed by not-so-bad weeks (as one mother of twins born at 26 weeks put it). Parents often worry that their feelings, about their baby and each other, are crazy, or that everyone expects them to handle their emotions better than they are doing. As we have emphasized throughout this book, everyone reacts and copes differently. However, we do want to share with you some of the feelings you may experience, and ways you might deal with them. The following paragraph is from a neonatologist who has worked with many premature infants and their parents; she is, moreover, the mother of a young child—born after she had spent several weeks on bedrest.

Many parents of premature infants feel, at some time, guilty, angry, afraid, sad, or just numb. Even with a healthy premature baby, you may feel disappointed at missing out on special plans you had made for your delivery or home-coming. Women who have to leave their babies in the hospital sometimes say that when they get home, they don't feel as if they had a baby. After months of visiting her baby in the intensive-care unit, one mother told me she still didn't feel like her little girl's mother. Someone else was always taking care of her baby. That experience is both the good side and the bad side of intensive care. On the one hand, it is reassuring to know that there is always a highly skilled person near your baby's bedside able to perform the complicated medical and nursing tasks needed. On the other hand, because the staff seems so competent, it is sometimes difficult for you to step in and help take care of your baby—especially if she is sick. However, it is important that you make the effort to get to know your baby while she is in the hospital, and to help care for her, when possible, by changing and bathing her, feeding her once she can take the bottle or the breast, and learning how to soothe her when she's upset. As you look around the room at all the experts who take care of your baby, remember you are her parents, the most important people in that room to your baby.

It's difficult to feel warm and motherly or fatherly when you are worried, exhausted, and under pressure. Sometimes, if your baby is very small or critically ill, the thought that she might die may make it too painful to become too involved with her. Even if the baby is doing well, you may not always feel maternal or paternal. Fatigue and worry (medical and/or financial) can make the situation more difficult. When your baby is born prematurely, you have missed much of the last weeks of pregnancy—a time most people spend preparing emotionally and physically to be new parents. However, getting to know your baby can help alleviate some of these feelings.

If you are uncomfortable touching the baby (a common reaction), just watch at first. See what she responds to, and how she responds. What does the baby like/dislike? Does she like having her head or back stroked, or does she seem more content when you just hold her hand? Babies recognize their mother's voice; when they're strong enough, babies will show they prefer it to all other voices. Even if your baby is too weak to respond, she may find your touch and voice comforting. Remember, tiny premature infants tire easily even from just listening or being stroked—so watch and learn how your baby looks when she is getting worn out. Soon you'll be the expert about your baby. Don't be afraid to share what you've noticed about your baby with the staff—how she responds, what seems to help. Your observations are important.

A word about "bonding," a term that has become popular in recent years. A baby born preterm may be whisked away to the NBICU shortly after birth. You may have only a few moments with him or her at most, right after delivery. If you have heard about "bonding" with your baby (spending time getting acquainted immediately after birth), you may wonder whether missing this particular time together will affect your feelings for each other later in life. Spending time with your baby right after birth is a wonderful experience, but it does not magically create an affectionate parent or a trusting and emotionally secure child. Those qualities develop with time. The emotional attachment that lets an infant develop trust in others and a sense of being loved and valued is learned throughout the first years of life—it is not determined in the first moments after birth.

Your lifelong relationship with your child can begin while your baby is in the nursery. Get to know your baby. Let her know that you are there, let her recognize your touch, the sound of your voice and the way you comfort her. Let the baby learn who her parents are, and who cares for her.

Prematurity—an Overview by Weeks

If your baby is born preterm, what can you expect? What will your baby look like? What health problems might she or he have?

It is important to realize that the preterm infant does not look or behave as the full-term baby does at birth. Depending upon the degree of prematurity, these differences may persist for weeks or even months after birth. Remember also that each baby is an individual with his or her own strengths and weaknesses. One baby born at 31 weeks' gestation may have medical problems that are quite different from another infant born at the same gestational age or having the same birth weight. While we cannot give you an exact description of your baby's medical course, we can give you some basic information about the most common problems preterm babies and their parents will encounter after birth.

You will see that potential complications are generally greater for babies born earlier; as a pregnancy progresses closer to 37 weeks, the likelihood of serious, long-lasting health problems declines. Every week really counts!

We will be concentrating primarily on gestational age— the number of weeks since your last menstrual period. Another very important factor is birth weight. Babies who weigh below normal range for their gestational age (at any stage of the pregnancy, even 37 weeks) are more susceptible to health problems than they would otherwise be. A nutritious diet throughout your pregnancy will pay off for your baby at the moment of birth!

A First Question: "Will My Baby Live?"

The fetus's physical features are formed by 16 weeks' gestation. The arms, legs, fingers, toes, ears, eyes, nose, and mouth are all present. The internal organs are formed, but require much more development before they can function independently of the mother's body. The second and third trimesters of pregnancy are a time of rapid physical growth for the fetus—laying down more muscle, bone, and fat, and gradually readying the body for life outside the womb. When this maturation process is interrupted by preterm delivery, the baby may not be able to perform all the body functions necessary for life. It may need outside help with these functions—help provided by the medical support of an intensive-care nursery.

With rare exceptions, infants born at or before 24 weeks' gestation are not mature enough to survive outside the womb, in spite of intensive life-support efforts in the nursery. You should be aware, however, that complex ethical and legal issues can arise regarding the treatment of these extremely premature infants. Decisions about what is best for your baby may be made by other people, and medical efforts may proceed even though the likelihood of death or of serious and permanent damage is very high. Premature infants born at the critical time, around 24 to 26 weeks, present a major dilemma to parents and medical and nursing personnel—technology may prolong life, or even result in survival, but with significant damage.

Infants born at 25 or 26 weeks of gestation (or any baby weighing less than 2 pounds) have about a 50 percent chance of surviving. With a few more weeks inside the womb, the baby's chances of living increase dramatically: close to 90 percent of babies born at 30 weeks will survive (*see figure 27*). Nevertheless, they must stay in the hospital for weeks, and in many cases for months, before they can go home.

The following section describes how your baby will probably look and act if a preterm birth cannot be avoided. We then discuss the most common medical problems of premature infants.

The Appearance and Behavior of Premature Infants

If born between 25 and 30 weeks of pregnancy: The average baby born at 25 weeks' gestation weighs about 1 pound, 10 ounces (750 grams) and is 13 inches long. By 30 weeks'

The Premature Infant

Gestational Age (in weeks)	Approximate Average Birth Weight	Survival
24	1 lb 4 oz (650 grams)	17%
26	2 lb (900 grams)	51%
28	2 lb 8 oz (1150 grams)	75%
30	3 lb 1 oz (1400 grams)	87%
32	3 lb 14 oz (1750 grams)	95%
34	4 lb 14 oz (2200 grams)	98%
36	5 lb 12 oz (2600 grams)	99+%

(Adapted from Goldenberg et al, *Obstetrics and Gynecology,* October 1984.)

Figure 27 — The premature infant.

gestation, the average weight is about 3 pounds (or 1350 grams), and the average length is about 15 inches. The weight of newborns does vary, depending upon the mother's size, diet, and health. An infant born at 25 weeks' gestation, for example, may weigh as little as 1 pound, 4 ounces (600 grams) and still be considered a normal weight for that gestational age.

Since most of the baby's fat supplies are laid down during the third trimester (the last 12 weeks or so of a full-term pregnancy), your baby will appear thin rather than pudgy like the full-term newborn. His fingers and toes will appear very long and slender, with tiny, completely formed fingernails and toenails. Because of the lack of fat beneath the skin, and the immaturity of the skin itself, it seems as if you can see right through the baby's skin. Tiny veins are seen easily through the skin, and the baby will usually be a ruddy red color at first, regardless of your ethnic background. The thin skin and lack of insulating fat layer means the baby does not yet have the usual built-in protection from chilling—he can become cold very easily, so he will be dried off quickly at birth, then kept bundled up, and warmed under special heat lamps or in a temperature-controlled incubator called an *isolette*. The baby will stay here until he has grown large enough to keep warm without extra help. Usually, a baby can maintain his own temperature—that is, keep warm enough—when he weighs about 4 pounds.

At birth, a thick, white, greasy substance—called *vernix*— can be seen on the baby's skin. This protective covering begins to appear between 17 and 20 weeks' gestation, and gradually decreases until term, when it is generally found only in the skin creases and the hair. The earlier the baby is born, the more completely covered he is with vernix.

In addition to the hair on his head, your baby will probably have fetal hair—called *lanugo*—on his face, shoulders, back, and perhaps his arms and legs. This body hair will gradually fall out as the baby matures, and will probably have disappeared by your due date.

At 25 to 28 weeks' gestation, your baby may not yet be able to cry loudly. He will sleep nearly 98 percent of the time. By 28 to 29 weeks' gestation, he may awaken fleetingly for a few seconds or a minute at a time. By this age, he may be capable of a weak cry. Returning to sleep may be difficult for the 28- to 29-week infant, and his sleep will seem restless, full of jerks, twitches, and facial movements (including smiles). This pattern of sleep is normal for a very premature infant. As he matures he will have longer periods of quiet sleep until his sleep pattern is more like that of an infant born at term— sleeping 75 percent of the time, with about half-quiet sleep and half-active sleep.

In contrast to activity while asleep, your baby may show little movement when awake. His muscle tone is not yet well developed, and he becomes exhausted easily. He may lie limply on his bed and offer little resistance when someone moves him. When a baby of this age does move, it is often with jerks and tremors. He has some normal reflex activity, such as sucking and swallowing (though these are not yet coordinated), grasping your finger when placed in his hand, showing a "startle response" to loud noise or to sudden movement of his body. He can sense the world around him—hear sounds, see light, and feel painful or pleasant touch against his skin. However, he is still too immature to react to these sensations in the same way a full-term baby would. For example, instead of opening his eyes, becoming quiet, or turning toward a sound, you may see only a change in heart rate, breathing, or skin color in response to stimulation. He can hear, see, and feel, but cannot yet physically organize a reaction, or behavior, that we can easily recognize.

In a full-term infant, we can often tell when the baby looks tired; in these very premature infants, however, we do not see the same signs. We do know that too much stimulation from outside can exhaust their energy very quickly. They are using their energy constantly to maintain a steady physical state. So be sure to talk with the nursing and medical staff about how much—or how little—touching or stroking seems best for your baby.

If born between 31 and 33 weeks of pregnancy: By 31 weeks' gestational age, your baby will be bigger, and probably healthier, at birth. The average baby at 31 weeks' gestation weighs about 3 pounds, 5 ounces (1500 grams) and is 16 inches long. Your baby at 31 weeks may weigh as little as 2 pounds, 7 ounces (1100 grams) or as much as 4 pounds, 5 ounces (1950 grams) and still be within the normal range. By 33 weeks' gestation she may weigh between 2 pounds, 15$\frac{1}{2}$ ounces (1350 grams) and 5 pounds, 5 ounces (2400 grams). The average is 3 pounds, 15$\frac{1}{2}$ ounces (1800 grams) and approximately 17$\frac{1}{2}$ inches in length. Survival rates for babies born during these weeks of pregnancy range from 90 to 98 percent. However, if your baby is born at 31 weeks' gestation, you should be prepared for her to remain hospitalized for perhaps five to eight weeks (depending on the possible medical problems) before she is ready to go home.

At 31 weeks' gestation your baby looks quite different than she did six weeks ago. Her skin is much less fragile. She now looks pink or ruddy red and her skin doesn't have that see-through look any more. She has more muscle and fat, but is still not chubby like the full-term infant. She cannot yet keep warm without extra heat from an incubator or heat lamp. Her head still seems large for her body and is heavy for her to move. She sleeps most of the time.

By now, though, the baby is stronger. In most cases, she can be touched and stroked for short periods of time without having changes in breathing, heart rate, or color. She moves more, and her muscles and reflexes—including grasping your hand—are stronger. She saves energy by sleeping a lot, and tires out very quickly after being touched, or changed, or examined by the doctors. She is not yet coordinated enough to suck from a bottle.

By 33 weeks' gestational age, she will be stronger and more active. Her skin color and breathing will be more stable, and she will tire less quickly. But sometimes, even if she is worn out after being excited, she has a hard time getting back to sleep or lying still and resting. Her body can move before she has developed the ability to control and quiet her waving arms and shaking legs. (You can sometimes help her calm down by gently holding her arms and legs close to her body.)

If born between 34 and 37 weeks of pregnancy: At 34 weeks' gestation, babies generally weigh between 3 pounds, 6 1/2 ounces (1550 grams) and 6 pounds, 3 ounces (2800 grams). The average weight is 4 pounds, 10 ounces (2100 grams), and the average length is 18 inches. At 37 weeks, babies weigh between 4 pounds, 13 1/2 ounces (2200 grams) and 7 pounds, 8 ounces (3400 grams); the average is 6 pounds, 3 ounces (2800 grams). Average length is about 19 inches. Survival rates at these gestational ages are over 99 percent. If the baby is not sick, his hospital stay may be very short—as little as one or two weeks for some 34-week infants, and just a few days for a healthy 37-week baby. Keep in mind, though, that before 37 complete weeks of pregnancy, your baby is more likely to have some problems associated with prematurity than if born a few weeks later.

A baby born at 34 or 35 weeks looks like a smaller, more slender version of a full-term baby. His skin is pink and soft. His hair is fluffy and fuzzy. His arms and legs have strength and more muscle tone, so he lies with his legs pulled up under him and offers more resistance to being moved. His reflexes are stronger. He can usually cry loudly enough to be heard, though he probably isn't strong enough to keep crying for more than a minute or two until close to 37 weeks.

When your baby wakes up, he now looks around and is even able to focus briefly on your face if it is nearby. By 37 to 38 weeks, if you move your face slowly while he is looking, he will follow you with his eyes. He will still tire easily, even after very pleasant times of being held and looking at you. Remember, he works very hard at staying awake, and concentrating and looking at you. By now, he can sometimes show you when he is worn out—by looking around, yawning, arching his back (rather than just "collapsing" from exhaustion, as a less mature infant does).

His movements are now more controlled, though still not as smooth and competent as the term baby's. His neck muscles are still weak, but by 36 to 37 weeks you can see him trying to lift his head up. By then he has enough control to cuddle up to you when you hold him instead of passively lying in your arms. Like less mature infants, he still cannot stay awake for long periods of time, and he often has a hard time waking up or going to sleep. His cues about what he needs ("I'm tired, I'm hungry, I'm wet") are not as easy to read as in a full-term infant. But before very long, you'll know!

Medical Problems of Premature Infants

We now turn to a brief overview of the most common medical problems seen in premature infants. The general types of illnesses described are similar for premature infants born at any gestational age. However, these conditions are usually more common and more serious in babies born very early and/or at a very low birth weight. We do *not* want the following discussion to upset or scare you. We *do* hope to provide you with basic information about problems your baby could develop, at different stages, if a preterm delivery occurs. This information may contribute to your decisions about treatment of preterm labor, may help you "stick it out" if, for example, you are on bedrest, and may be useful to you *if* your baby is premature.

First we describe the medical problems as they commonly

appear in the *most* susceptible infants—those born *between 25 and 30 weeks* of pregnancy. After this introduction, we'll discuss how these conditions generally change—becoming less frequent and less severe—in babies born closer to term.

Respiratory Distress Syndrome (RDS)

Respiratory distress syndrome (*RDS*), also called *hyaline membrane disease* (*HMD*), is the most common breathing disorder found in premature infants. The lung has tiny air sacs (*alveoli*) where oxygen (O_2) is taken into the bloodstream and carbon dioxide (CO_2) is given off to be exhaled. To accomplish this task efficiently, the alveoli must remain slightly inflated at all times, and not collapse like an empty balloon at the end of each breath. The body makes a substance called *surfactant*, which coats the alveoli, preventing their collapse while still allowing exchange of oxygen and carbon dioxide.

The fetus begins to make surfactant early in pregnancy, but there is usually not enough surfactant for smooth and easy breathing until 35 weeks' gestation. Babies vary a great deal in the amount of surfactant made, and how well their lungs work, at any particular gestational age. Nearly all infants weighing less than 1000 grams or born at less than 30 weeks' gestation will need treatment for breathing difficulties of RDS. A smaller percentage of older, larger infants, and even a very few full-term infants, can also be affected by RDS, some severely, others mildly. A physical stress such as difficult delivery, chilling the body, or low oxygen levels in the baby's blood, can increase the risk of developing RDS.

The type of treatment depends on the baby's needs. Your baby may require only some extra oxygen to breathe. Oxygen can be pumped into the enclosed beds (*isolettes*) or delivered into a clear plastic bubble (called a *hood*) placed over a baby's head. If your baby is weaker, or needs more concentrated amounts of oxygen, she may be given additional help with breathing. A mask is placed over her mouth and nose, or a soft, flexible nosepiece fitted into her nostrils, giving "continuous positive airway pressure" (CPAP), which reduces the physical effort your baby must provide to inflate collapsed air sacs with each breath.

Many infants born between 24 and 30 weeks' gestation require *intubation* to be sure the actual breathing process occurs regularly. A flexible plastic tube about the diameter of your baby's finger, called an *endotracheal (ET) tube*, is inserted through her nose or mouth and positioned in the windpipe (*trachea*). The ET tube can deliver the needed oxygen *and* be connected to a breathing machine (*ventilator*), providing mechanical breaths that are more efficient than the baby's own weak and often irregular respirations.

If your child is receiving supplemental oxygen, the doctors need to know how much oxygen is actually getting into the blood. One type of oxygen-measure is through a dime-sized heated sensor placed onto the baby's skin which gives a continuous reading of oxygen levels in the bloodstream. Periodically, blood samples will be taken to measure the oxygen, carbon dioxide, and acid (pH) levels in her blood. These samples can sometimes be collected through a small tube (called a *catheter*) placed directly into the umbilical artery and threaded from there into the aorta, the main blood vessel supplying oxygenated blood to the body. The tube can be placed without discomfort and allows continuous monitoring of blood pressure, as well as painless withdrawal of blood and administration of fluid. These umbilical artery (UA) catheters can be used for only a short time after birth; later on, blood samples are taken either by pricking the baby's heel (*heelstick*) or by drawing directly with a very small needle from an artery or vein.

Patent Ductus Arteriosus (PDA)

Your baby's blood circulates differently while he is still in the womb than after he is born. Before birth, oxygen is taken into his bloodstream directly from your placenta without use of the lungs. The blood circulation detours away from his unused lungs to the rest of his body through a blood vessel called the *ductus arteriosus* (*see figure 28*). When the baby starts breathing at birth this special "detour" channel must close so that the lungs can function in the outside world. If this ductus does not close, oxygenated (bright red) blood that has passed through the lungs once and is ready to be pumped

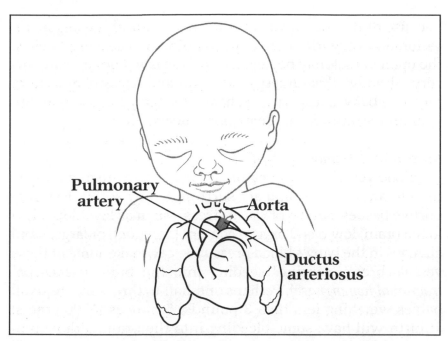

Figure 28 — Neonatal circulation with a patent ductus arteriosus.

to the body flows instead through the open channel—the "patent" ductus arteriosus (PDA)—and floods into the lungs a second time. This extra blood then flows from the lungs back into the left side of the heart again, overloading it and making it pump less effectively. This condition can develop into congestive heart failure. PDA is a common problem in premature infants because their bodies have not had time before birth to close this special vessel, a process that normally occurs at term. In some cases, PDAs may close and then reopen, triggered by physical stresses such as breathing difficulties, too much fluid retention in the circulation, or other problems.

There are several treatments for PDAs, depending upon how ill the baby is. The simplest treatment, often effective for larger babies, is to limit the fluid given the baby; this reduces the work the overloaded heart must do. For babies born at less than 30 weeks' gestation, this technique alone is usually not enough. A medication called indomethacin may also be needed. This medicine can trigger the baby's PDA-closing mechanism; it is effective in some cases but the effects may not last. Nor can indomethacin be used in all babies because of its side effects. If reducing fluids and using medication do not work or are not possible, then surgery to close the open vessel may be necessary. This is *not* open heart surgery. Although this surgery is a serious and stressful procedure for a tiny baby, in experienced hands the baby tolerates surgery well and strain on the heart is reduced.

Intracranial Hemorrhage (ICH)

Blood vessels in a premature infant's brain are more fragile than in a term baby, and are surrounded by softer, less supportive tissues. Severe physical stress—such as low blood flow to the brain, low blood oxygen content (*asphyxia*), or large, rapid changes in the baby's blood pressure—can make some of these vessels break, causing bleeding into the brain tissues (*intracranial hemorrhage*). Perhaps one-half to three-fourths of all babies weighing less than 3 pounds, 5 ounces (1500 grams) at birth will have some bleeding into the brain, although in most babies the amount is very small. The more mature and healthly the baby is at birth, the less likely she is to have bleeding problems. The effect of intracranial bleeding on a baby's present or future health and brain function depends on the amount and location of bleeding, as well as on the severity of the physical stress causing the bleeding.

Intracranial hemorrhage can be diagnosed in two ways. One method uses a special computerized x-ray device, called a *C.T.* or *C.A.T. scanner*. The scan produces a picture of the brain itself, including the normal fluid-filled sacs (*ventricles*) and any abnormal bleeding. This procedure can usually be done without discomfort to the baby, though the baby must be moved to the machine. A second diagnostic method uses an ultrasound scanner to detect bleeding (this type of machine, which uses sound waves rather than x-rays, may have been used during pregnancy to measure your baby's size, position, or the position of the placenta in the womb). The ultrasound scanner can be used at your baby's bedside.

If an intracranial hemorrhage is discovered, the baby will be watched carefully. The bleeding itself must heal on its own since there is no treatment. Although most babies will have small bleeds that have no long-term consequences, complications can develop in a small number of cases.

Infection

The preterm infant is more vulnerable to infection than a term baby. His infection-fighting immune system is less mature, and he has not yet had the chance to build up resistance to infections. He does get some infection-fighting proteins, called *antibodies*, from the mother's bloodstream before birth, but his resistance is still low. If an illness develops, resistance may be further weakened.

In older children the immune system quickly confines infection to one body system—lungs, skin, throat, etc. Clear signals of infection appear, such as fever, sore throat, high white blood cell count. Because an infant's immune system is not yet fully working, infection is more likely to affect many areas at once; germs can spread rapidly, and the usual signs of bacteria may not be apparent. Therefore, when infection is suspected, all body systems—lungs, blood, urine, and especially brain—are tested for the presence and extent of infection. Since infections can be very serious in a newborn infant, antibiotics are started as soon as the tests are done; if the test results show no infection after several days, the antibiotics may be stopped.

Intensive-care nurseries and well-baby nurseries take precautions to protect babies from unnecessary exposure to germs. The hospital staff will probably remind you to wash your hands thoroughly before entering, and to wear a gown over your street clothes. If you have a fever, cold, sore throat, flu, or cold sore, check with your baby's doctor about visiting and about extra precautions you should take.

Feeding and Fluids

Babies younger than 34 weeks' gestation are often not yet able to take their feedings directly from the bottle or breast; sucking, swallowing, and breathing are not yet synchronized. To prevent the baby from getting milk "down the wrong pipe" into his lungs, he will be fed through a *nasogastric (NG) tube*. This tube is passed through his nose or mouth into his stomach and formula or breast milk is dripped through the tube in tiny amounts. The tube is removed after each feeding. When the baby is able to breathe comfortably while eating, using a feeding tube is no longer necessary.

A baby who has been very physically stressed may need to rest and recover his digestive system before he can accept milk or formula. Until he can be fed either by mouth or even with an NG tube, he will need to receive fluids, minerals, sugar (glucose), and other nutrients through blood veins. The amounts of water, salts, sugar, and protein given intravenously must be measured very carefully to assure that his body is handling them correctly. A premature infant's kidneys do not work as efficiently as an adult's, or even as well as a full-term infant's. Because the premature infant cannot regulate water, salt, and waste products quickly, intake and urine output will be measured and blood level of salts monitored closely.

The amount of blood required for various tests is quite small; however, many tests may be needed, and premature infants cannot make new red blood cells rapidly enough to replace those removed for blood tests. Premature babies are also low in iron because most iron is transferred from mother to baby during the 28th to 40th week of pregnancy. To avoid anemia (low amounts of red blood cells and the iron they carry), premature infants often need blood transfusions.

Remember: The medical problems described occur mainly in the most premature newborns. Things begin to look better in babies born after 30 weeks' gestation (*see figure 29*).

If born between 31 and 33 weeks of pregnancy: Your baby is still likely to have some problems with respiratory distress syndrome, patent ductus arteriosus, and possibly with intracranial hemorrhage or infection (described in the previous section). However, babies born at this stage of a pregnancy are usually not so sick as smaller, more premature babies. They experience fewer complications and recover more quickly from medical problems that do develop.

Apnea is a breathing problem that can arise among infants who are breathing on their own (that is, they do not require a mechanical respirator). Apnea means an abnormally long pause in the baby's breathing, lasting 20 seconds or more.

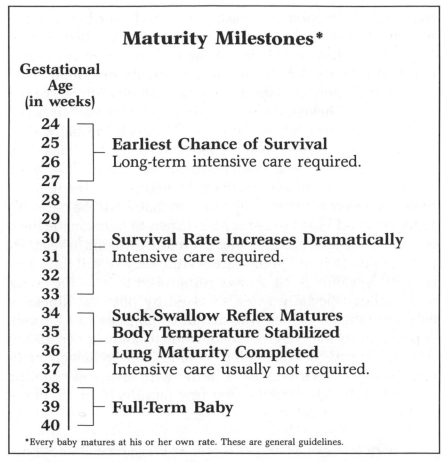

Figure 29 — Maturity milestones.

Many premature infants have short pauses where they stop breathing for five to 10 seconds followed by at least 10 to 15 seconds of fast breathing. During these five- to 10-second pauses, the baby's skin color and heart rate usually don't change. If the baby stops breathing for 20 seconds or more (an *apneic spell*), his skin color changes as his blood oxygen level falls, and his heart beat slows to an abnormally low rate. He may start breathing again on his own or he may need to be aroused and reminded to breathe by being firmly patted or rubbed. Occasionally this kind of stimulation isn't enough to restart normal breathing. Then the nurse will give him mechanical breaths by squeezing a soft inflatable bag filled with oxygen and attached to a mask positioned over his nose and mouth. Breathing for the baby in this way is called *bagging*.

If the medical staff is not at the bedside, they are alerted to a change in the baby's condition by an alarm system called a *monitor*. A monitor uses special pads stuck onto the baby's skin to detect heart rate and respirations. If these fall below normal, an alarm warns the nurse to check the baby.

Babies may have apnea for many reasons. Low blood oxygen or high blood acid content (*acidosis*), low levels of sugar or calcium in the blood, seizures, or infection in the lungs or bloodstream can all cause apnea. The baby will be carefully examined and blood tests may be drawn to help decide what is causing the apnea. Sometimes premature infants have apnea just because they are premature. While they're still tiny, their nervous systems don't always remember to give the signal to breathe, especially when stressed by physical illness or extreme fatigue. Babies who are having apnea just because of prematurity may be given medication to stimulate breathing. As they mature, their breathing becomes more reliable. Rarely, there is a need to send a baby home with an apnea monitor, which will be used for the first few months of life to check on the baby's breathing.

If born between 34 and 37 weeks of pregnancy: Babies born between 34 and 37 weeks' gestation are much *less* likely to have serious problems with respiratory distress syndrome (RDS), infections, or intracranial hemorrhage (ICH) (described earlier in this chapter). They may have some milder breathing problems, and usually need some time before they are able to feed and gain weight well. It may take them longer than a full-term infant for them to nurse effectively. They generally do not require as much mechanical assistance as babies born earlier. The larger infants of this 34- to 37-week group are often able to regulate their own body temperature; smaller infants, however, may still need help, for instance from heating lamps.

Jaundice of the newborn is a problem that can arise in preterm and full-term infants. It is commonly treated by use of special lights (*phototherapy*).

If you are a high-risk pregnant woman who is approaching the 34th or 35th week of pregnancy, you can let yourself feel good. The risks associated with prematurity are definitely reduced, and before *too* long, you will be "at term."

Congratulations!

A P P E N D I X

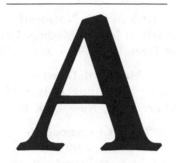

Resource
List

Books

Brown, J. E. *Nutrition for Your Pregnancy: The University of Minnesota Guide.* Minneapolis: University of Minnesota Press, 1983.

DES Action. *Fertility and Pregnancy Guide for DES Daughters and Sons.* New Hyde Park, New York: DES Action National, 1983.

Friedman, R., and Gradstein, B. *Surviving Pregnancy Loss.* Boston: Little, Brown, and Company, 1982.

Harrison, H. *The Premature Baby Book.* New York: St. Martin's Press, 1983.

Gill, P., and Katz, M. *Let's Prevent Preterm Birth* (pamphlet). Santa Ana, California: Tokos Medical Corporation, 1985.

Gill, P., Smith, M., Katz, M. *Tocolysis for Preterm Labor* (pamphlet). Santa Ana, California: Tokos Medical Corporation, 1987.

Robertson, P. A., and Berlin, P. H. *The Premature Labor Handbook.* New York: Doubleday and Company, Inc., 1986.

Smith, M., Gill, P., and Katz, M. *The Premature Baby* (pamphlet). Santa Ana, California: Tokos Medical Corporation, 1987.

Medically Oriented Books

Fuchs, F., and Stubblefield, P. G. (eds.). *Preterm Birth: Causes, Prevention and Management*, New York: Macmillan Publishing Company, 1984.

Worthington-Roberts, B. S., Vermeersch, J., and Williams, S. R. *Nutrition in Pregnancy and Lactation*, 2nd ed. St. Louis: C.V. Mosby Company, 1981.

Organizations

DES Action National
Long Island Jewish Medical Center
New Hyde Park, New York 11040

March of Dimes
1275 Mamaroneck Avenue
White Plains, New York 10605

Triplet Connection
P.O. Box 99571
Stockton, California 95209

Twin Line
P.O. Box 10066
Berkeley, California 94709

APPENDIX

B

A
Relaxation
Technique*

Have someone with a soothing voice read the following directions for relaxation to you or prepare a tape recording to assist you in practicing.

Open your mouth wide as you inhale and sigh out the breath: a-a-a-h. Repeat five times.

Focus your concentration on your facial muscles and feel the forehead and eyebrow area going limp. Make that area let go even more.

Mentally focus on your eyes. Relax your eyes.

Feel your jaw muscles and cheek muscles let go. Feel the looseness. Separate your teeth and let your tongue fall back slightly into your mouth. Feel the muscles in the mouth area letting go.

Feel your nostrils, ears, and scalp relaxing.

Let all expression melt from your face. Feel it going limp.

---

*Adapted from *Positive Pregnancy Fitness* by Sylvia Klein Olkin. Used with permission of the author.

Relax the neck: the front, the sides, the back of the neck.

Feel your shoulders letting go: the right shoulder, the left shoulder, and the space between.

Feel your upper arms, elbows, lower arms relaxing.

Feel your fingers opening slightly and releasing.

Feel your chest and back going limp. Feel the top half of your body completely relaxed and loose.

Relax the tummy area to give the baby more room. Feel the inner abdominal muscles letting go.

Feel your buttocks going limp, letting go.

Focus in on the birth canal area and feel it become loose and relaxed. Check to see that your mouth is still relaxed. Relax the mouth and the birth canal.

Feel your thighs, hips, knees, calves, and ankles going limp. Feel your feet letting go. Make your toes relax one by one.

Take a moment or two to check your body over for further tension.

Feel yourself sinking into the bed. Let go, give up. Feel a sense of looseness enveloping you.

Feel the tensions draining out of your fingers and your toes. Imagine a flow of tensions, tiredness, troubles, fears, anxieties, and aches leaving your body as you open all the muscles.

Let your breathing settle down to a comfortable rate as you sink into the blissful feeling of complete relaxation.

Try to keep your mental awareness on how your body feels. Become aware of your hands and legs. Move your fingers slowly, then your toes, then begin to stretch and slowly arouse.

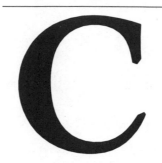

Shopping
by
Mail

General

Sears, J.C. Penney, Best Consumer's Distributing (check your phone book for these stores or their catalog offices).

Maternity and Nursing Clothes

Easy Feed, Inc., P.O. Box 35238, Phoenix, AZ, 85069; nursing clothes. Send stamped, self-addressed envelope.

Practical Elegance, 200 Gate 5 Road, Suite 203, Sausalito, CA 94965; maternity and nursing lingerie.

5th Ave. Maternity, P.O. Box 21826, Seattle WA, 98111.

Infant Clothing, Furniture, Supplies, Toys

After the Stork, P.O. Box 4488, Albuquerque, NM 89196; toys, clothes.

Baby News: Check your telephone book for any store with "Baby News" in its name, and phone for its very complete catalog.

Baby Toytown, 800-423-3368 (in California), 8938 E. Valley Blvd., Rosemead, CA 91770.

INDEX

Adrenalin, 87
Alcohol, 15, 19, 95-96
Amniocentesis, 108
Anesthesia
  during forceps delivery, 115
  for episiotomy, 116
  regional, 114
Apnea, 136-38
Asphyxia, 134

Bathing
  during bedrest, 67, 70
  while hospitalized, 107
Bedrest, 16, 51-77, 106
  childbirth preparation during, 71
  child care during, 63-65
  emotions about, 55-61
  exercise during, 60, 68-69, 71
  financial aid during, 64, 71-72
  getting up from, 53
  household help during, 62-63
  insomnia during, 69-70
  nutrition during, 73-74, 75-77
  organizing for, 61-62
  outings during, 71
  prescribing, 51
  resources during, 62-63, 64, 73, 143-44
  shopping during, 70-71, 147
  things to do during, 66-68
  things to have during, 65-66
  to stop preterm labor, 16, 45, 47
  types of, 52, 54
Beta-adrenergics (Beta-mimetics)
  administering, 88-90
  described, 87-88
  measuring pulse rate while on, 88-89, 90
  side effects of
    on baby, 92-93
    on pregnant woman, 90-92
  taking pulse while on, 101-102
Betamethasone, 97, 105
Beta-mimetics. See Beta-adrenergics.
Bladder
  control while working, 17
  emptying, 107
  full as false contractions, 42
Blood
  pressure changes

  in baby, 93
  in pregnant woman, 98
  sugar levels in baby, 92, 93
  tests, while hospitalized, 108
Bonding, 123-24
Braxton-Hicks contractions, 33, 35
Breast stimulation, 18
Breathing
  disorders in baby, 131-34, 136-37
  during pregnancy. See Exercise.
Breech birth, 114, 115
Brethine, 87
Bricanyl, 87

Calcium
  deficiency in baby, 93, 95
  entry blockers, 96-97
Cerclage, 79-84
  described, 79-82
  timing of, 82
  weighing risks and benefits of, 83-84
Cervical incompetence, 40, 79, 80
Cervix
  changes in
    during labor, 40
    early detection of, 48
    limiting exercise after, 18
    as sign of labor, 8
  dilation of, 40, 79
  effacement of, 40
  incompetence in. See Cervical incompetence.
Cesarean delivery
  after abdominal cerclage, 82
  during preterm delivery, 113-14
Colase, 102
Constipation
  bedrest as cause of, 74
  regulating, with food intake, 76-77
  tocolytic medications and, 102
Contractions
  Braxton-Hicks, 33, 35
  detecting, 30-32, 35-36, 44
  during labor, 39
  during preterm labor, 28-29
  false, 42
  pain and, 35
  recording, with home electronic monitor, 104